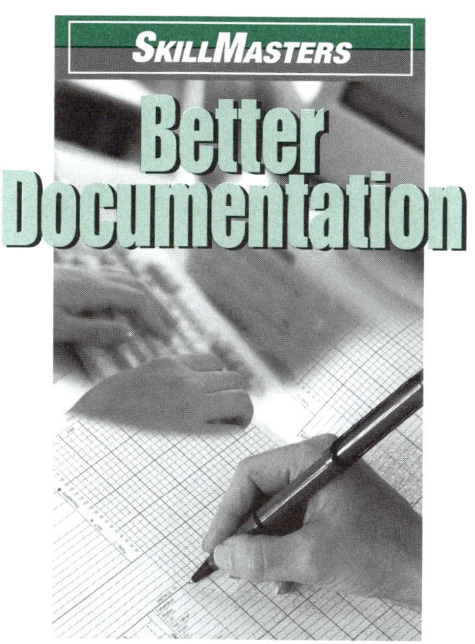
SKILLMASTERS
Better
Documentation

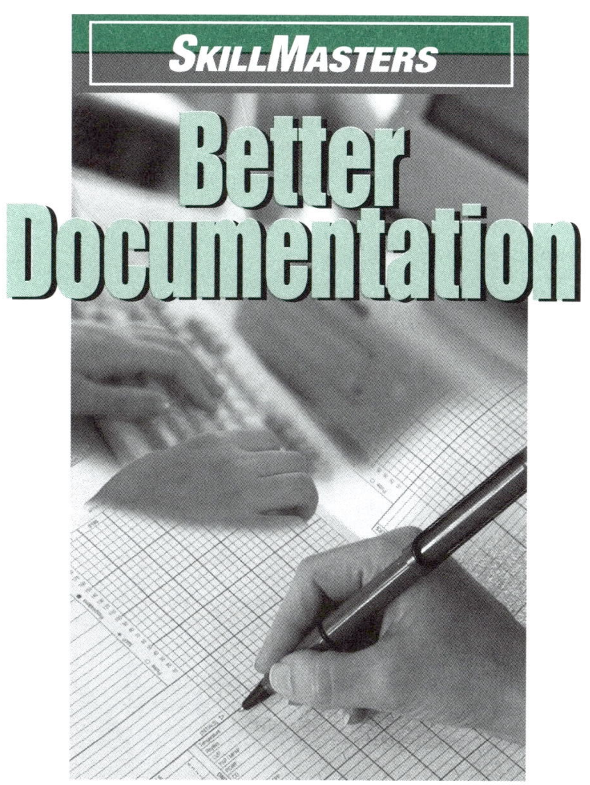

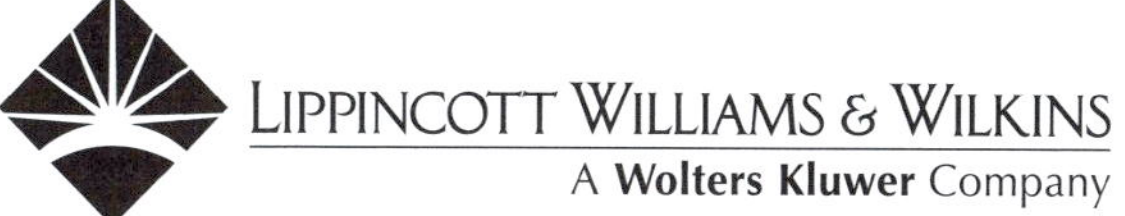

Lippincott Williams & Wilkins
A **Wolters Kluwer** Company
Philadelphia • Baltimore • New York • London
Buenos Aires • Hong Kong • Sydney • Tokyo

Staff

Publisher
Judith A. Schilling McCann, RN, MSN

Editorial Director
H. Nancy Holmes

Clinical Director
Joan M. Robinson, RN, MSN

Senior Art Director
Arlene Putterman

Clinical Editor
Jana L. Sciarra (clinical project manager), RN, MSN, CRNP

Editors
Jennifer P. Kowalak (senior associate editor)

Copy Editors
Kimberly Bilotta, Heather Ditch, Dolores Matthews, Dorothy Terry, Peggy Williams

Designers
Mary Ludwicki (art director), BJ Crim (book designer), Lynn Foulk

Cover Design
Risa Clow, Robert Dieters

Electronic Production Services
Diane Paluba (manager), Joyce Rossi Biletz (senior desktop assistant), Richard Eng

Manufacturing
Patricia K. Dorshaw (senior manager), Beth Janae Orr (book production coordinator)

Editorial Assistants
Danielle J. Barsky, Carol Caputo, Beverly Lane, Linda Ruhf

Librarian
Catherine M. Heslin

Indexer
Karen C. Comerford

The clinical treatments described and recommended in this publication are based on research and consultation with nursing, medical, and legal authorities. To the best of our knowledge, these procedures reflect currently accepted practice. Nevertheless, they can't be considered absolute and universal recommendations. For individual applications, all recommendations must be considered in light of the patient's clinical condition and, before administration of new or infrequently used drugs, in light of the latest package-insert information. The authors and publisher disclaim any responsibility for any adverse effects resulting from the suggested procedures, from any undetected errors, or from the reader's misunderstanding of the text.

 Printed in the United States of America. For information, write Lippincott Williams & Wilkins, 1111 Bethlehem Pike, P.O. Box 908, Springhouse, PA 19477-0908.

SBD – D N O S A J J M A
05 04 03 10 9 8 7 6 5 4 3 2

Library of Congress Cataloging-in-Publication Data
Skillmasters : better documentation.
p. ; cm.
Includes index.
Nursing records — Handbooks, manuals, etc.
[DNLM: 1. Nursing Records. 2. Documentation — methods. 3. Forms and Records Control. WY 100.5 S628b 2003] I. Title: Better documentation. II. Lippincott Williams & Wilkins.
RT50 .S557 2003
651.5'04261—dc21
ISBN 1-58255-177-4 (phb. : alk. paper) 2002004446

Contents

Contributors and consultants **vii**
Foreword **ix**

Chapter 1 Fundamentals of documentation 1
Chapter 2 Legal aspects of documentation 51
Chapter 3 Documentation systems 62
Chapter 4 Documenting in acute care 93
Chapter 5 Documenting in long-term care 116
Chapter 6 Documenting in home care 138
Chapter 7 Documenting in special situations 156

Appendices
A. Commonly accepted abbreviations 188
B. Commonly accepted symbols 197
C. NANDA Taxonomy II codes 199
Selected references 202
Index 203

Contributors and consultants

Debra Aucoin-Ratcliff, RN, MN
Nursing Program Director
Western Career College
Sacramento, Calif.

Athena A. Foreman, RN, MSN
Nursing Coordinator
Stanley Community College
Albemarle, N.C.

Lisa A. Salamon, RN,C, MSN
Clinical Nurse Specialist
Cleveland Clinic Foundation

Lourdes "Cindy" Santoni-Reddy, RN, MSN, MEd, CPP, FAAPM, NP-C
Pain Management Practitioner
Researcher
CRNP Associates, P.C.
Yardley, Pa.

Pamela B. Simmons, RN, PhD
Assistant Hospital Administrator for Patient Care Services
Louisiana State University Health Sciences Center
Shreveport

Marilyn Smith-Stoner, RN, PhD
Adjunct Faculty
University of Phoenix (Ariz.)
Home Care Consultant
Ontario, Calif.

Catherine Ultrino, RN, MSN, OCN
Nurse Manager
Boston Medical Center

Marilyn J. Vontz, RN, PhD
Nurse Educator
Bryan Hospital School of Nursing
Lincoln, Nebr.

Suzanne P. Weaver, RN, RHIT, CPHQ
Director of Nursing
Neshaminy Manor
Warrington, Pa.

Foreword

Now as never before, with consumer and market-driven forces playing a greater role in health care delivery, it's crucial for nurses to have the skills required to produce accurate, effective, and efficient documentation.

To that end, it's essential that nurses have a reference guide on documentation that's easy to use and that covers fundamentals, legal aspects, special situations, and a variety of documentation systems for a variety of settings (acute care, long-term care, and home care). *SkillMasters: Better Documentation* is that reference guide.

Not only is documentation the main communication tool among professional health care team members, it's used to justify medical treatment and reimbursement and to satisfy regulatory, licensing, and accreditation requirements. Students, faculty and researchers, lawyers and judges, Medicare, Medicaid, and insurance companies as well as peer reviewers, and even an institution's own performance improvement team rely on documentation to fulfill the multiple demands of today's health care management. The more documentation is reviewed and used, the more critical that it be accurate and of the highest quality.

SkillMasters: Better Documentation provides guidelines for essentially every patient care setting in a variety of health care delivery systems. It also demonstrates efficient and effective documentation by giving the nurse sample forms that show exactly how to document nursing assessments, interventions, evaluations, and outcomes. Included are guidelines for using computerized documentation systems, traditional narrative documenting, problem-oriented medical records, the FOCUS system, the problem-intervention-evaluation system, charting by exception, and the FACT documentation system. Additionally, this fact-filled book discusses the advantages and disadvantages of each documentation system along with advice on how to choose an appropriate documentation system.

Highlighted throughout *SkillMasters: Better Documentation* are several time-saving techniques that can provide a more concise written record without sacrificing accuracy or legal protections. This valuable guidebook also gives pointers on how to identify legal hazards and avoid the possibility of a lawsuit. Legal standards of documentation, such as nurse practice acts, standards of the Joint Commission on Accreditation of Healthcare Organizations, and malpractice litigation, are discussed with tips on how to utilize risk management techniques.

Critical pathways, care plans, progress notes, activities of daily living checklists, flow sheets – all are discussed and demonstrated in *SkillMasters: Better Documentation.* Also shown in examples are the standardized and required documents used in long-term care and the Medicare-mandated forms needed in home care.

Another outstanding feature in *SkillMasters: Better Documentation* is the

SkillCheck at the end of each chapter. This self-quiz is designed to help nurses or nursing students practice and use what the chapter has discussed.

All in all, *SkillMasters: Better Documentation* offers a wealth of information, useful sample documentation forms, and self-help skills evaluation in every chapter. *SkillMasters: Better Documentation* leads the way to superior documentation and helps nurses demonstrate the quality and value of their nursing care.

Jacqueline Walus-Wigle, RN, JD, CPHQ
Manager of Compliance, Regulatory, and External Affairs
University of California, San Diego Healthcare

1 Fundamentals of documentation

Documentation — or charting — is the process of preparing a complete record of a patient's care. Accurate, detailed documentation shows the extent and quality of the care you've provided, the outcome of that care, and the treatment and education that the patient still needs.

Documentation is a vital tool for communication among health care team members. Frequently, decisions, actions, and revisions related to the patient's care are based on documentation from various team members. A well-prepared medical record shows the high degree of collaboration among health care team members.

The information that's documented by team members must be easily retrievable and readable because a patient's medical record may be read by a wide audience, including:

- other members of the health care team
- reviewers from accrediting, certifying, and licensing organizations
- performance-improvement monitors
- peer reviewers
- Medicare and insurance company reviewers
- researchers and teachers
- attorneys and judges.

Proper documentation is important for other reasons. One of the most compelling reasons for you to develop good documentation practices is to establish your professional responsibility and accountability.

In the past, documentation consisted of cursory observations, such as *patient ate well* or *patient slept well.* The chief purpose of these documents was to show that the physician's orders and the facility's policies had been followed and that the patient had received the proper care.

In the 19th century, British nurse Florence Nightingale paved the way for modern nursing documentation. In her book, *Notes on Nursing*, she stressed the importance of training nurses to gather patient information in a clear, concise, organized manner. As her theories gained acceptance, nurses' perceptions and observations about patient care gained credence and respect. More than a century later, in the 1970s, nurses began creating their own vocabulary for documentation based on nursing diagnoses.

Purposes of documentation

Accurate nursing documentation is important for many reasons, including these nine:

- It's a mode of communication among health care professionals.

- It's checked in health care evaluations.
- It's legal evidence that protects you.
- It's used to aid research and education.
- It helps facilities obtain accreditation and licenses.
- It's used to justify reimbursement requests.
- It's used to develop improvements in the quality of care.
- It indicates compliance with your nurse practice act.
- It establishes professional accountability.

COMMUNICATION

Patients receive care from many people who work different shifts, and these various caregivers may speak with each other infrequently. The medical record is the main source of information and communication among nurses, physicians, physical therapists, social workers, and other caregivers. Today, nurses are often considered managers of care as well as practitioners, and nurses usually document the most information. Everyone's notes are important, however, because together they present a complete picture of the patient's care.

As health care facilities continue to streamline and redesign care delivery systems, tasks that were historically performed by nurses are now being assigned to multiskilled workers. To deliver highly specialized care, each caregiver must provide accurate, thorough information and be able to interpret what others have written about a patient. Then each can use this information to plan future patient care.

HEALTH CARE EVALUATION

When health care is evaluated by other members of the health care team — reviewers, insurance companies, Medicare representatives, attorneys, or judges — accurate documentation is one way to prove that you're providing high-quality care. Complete documentation is both a record of what you do for your patient and written evidence that this care is necessary. It's also a record of your patient's response to your care and any changes you make in his care plan.

LEGAL PROTECTION

On the legal side, accurate documentation shows that the care you provide meets the patient's needs and expressed wishes. It also proves that you're following the accepted standards of nursing care mandated by the law, your profession, and your health care facility.

Proper documentation communicates crucial clinical information to caregivers so they make fewer errors. How and what you document can determine whether you or your employer wins or loses a legal dispute. Medical records are used as evidence in cases involving disability, personal injury, and mental competency. Poor documentation is the pivotal issue in many malpractice cases.

RESEARCH AND EDUCATION

Documentation also provides data for research and continuing education. For example, researchers and nurse educators may study medical records to determine the effectiveness of nursing care. Medical records may also be used to gauge how patient teaching affects compliance; the patient's educational level and barriers to learning are noted, as is an assessment of how well he followed the treatment regimen.

Just as documentation is used in research, research studies can be used to improve documentation practices. For example, studies may uncover errors in the medical record, thereby pointing out the need for continuing education programs for health care providers.

ACCREDITING AND LICENSING

For a facility to remain accredited, caregivers must document care that reflects the standards set by national organizations, such as the American Nurses Association and the Joint Commission on Accreditation of Healthcare Organizations (JCAHO). Some states also require facilities to be licensed; licensing laws, in turn, require each facility to establish policies and procedures for operation.

A facility's accreditation and licensure may be jeopardized by substandard documentation. When a facility is cited for having poor documentation or not meeting set standards, it receives a warning, and a target date is set for the facility to make necessary changes and corrections. A facility may lose its license if it doesn't carry out these actions.

In effect, accreditation is evidence that a facility provides quality care and is qualified to receive federal funds. The federal government works with state accrediting organizations to make sure facilities are eligible to receive Medicare reimbursement. Accreditation and reimbursement eligibility require documentation that accurately reflects the care provided to patients. Good documentation demonstrates that facility and state nursing policies were followed.

Officials of accrediting organizations look at a facility's structure and function to decide if the facility should be accredited. They also conduct surveys and audits of patient and medical records to see if care meets the required standards.

Officials review charts and files to ensure good documentation. For example, in a case in which physical restraints were used, officials may ask, "Is there a form for documenting the need for restraints and their correct use?" and, "Does the documentation in the charts show that restraints were used correctly?" Proper documentation reflects the quality of care provided and the facility's accountability.

Accrediting organizations also regularly survey and audit records to make sure the standard of care is consistent throughout a facility. For example, a woman recovering from anesthesia after a cesarean birth should expect to receive the same monitoring in the labor and delivery suite as she would in the postanesthesia care unit. JCAHO inspectors review the documentation of both departments to ensure that a uniform standard of care is given and documented. Most accrediting organizations have similar standards for documentation. (See *Components of the clinical record*, page 4.)

REIMBURSEMENT

Reimbursement from Medicare and insurance companies depends heavily on accurate nursing documentation. For example, many facilities today use elaborate electronic dispensing carts to keep track of supplies. To be reimbursed for these supplies, nursing documentation has to justify their use.

CHECKLIST

Components of the clinical record

Accrediting organizations require many of the same standards for documentation. For example, each patient's medical record must contain:

- ❑ identification data
- ❑ the medical history, which includes the patient's reason for seeking care; details of his present illness; relevant past, social, and family histories; and a body system assessment
- ❑ a summary of the patient's psychosocial needs as appropriate for his age
- ❑ a report of relevant physical examination findings
- ❑ a statement of the impressions drawn from the admission history and physical examination
- ❑ the care plan
- ❑ diagnostic and therapeutic orders
- ❑ evidence of informed consent
- ❑ clinical observations, including the effects of treatment
- ❑ progress notes
- ❑ consultation reports, if applicable
- ❑ reports of operative and other invasive procedures, tests, and their results, if appropriate
- ❑ reports of diagnostic and therapeutic procedures, such as radiology and nuclear medicine examinations
- ❑ records of donation and receipt of transplants or implants, if applicable
- ❑ a final diagnosis
- ❑ discharge summaries and instructions
- ❑ results of autopsy, when performed.

Meeting requirements

Some organizations spell out the information each of these forms must contain. In these cases, the nurse-manager must write and implement guidelines that meet these requirements.

Documentation is also used to determine the amount of reimbursement a facility receives. The federal government, for example, uses a prospective payment system based on diagnosis-related groups (DRGs) to determine Medicare reimbursements. In other words, it pays a fixed amount for a particular diagnosis. For a facility to receive payment, the patient's medical record at discharge must contain the correct DRG codes and show that he received the proper care, including appropriate patient teaching and discharge planning.

Most insurance companies also base reimbursements on a prospective payment system, and they usually don't reimburse for unskilled nursing care. They pay for skilled medical and nursing care only. For example, they compensate nurse practitioners and home health care nurses for skilled care, which includes assessing a patient's condition, creating a care plan, and following a strict treatment regimen.

Before reimbursing, an examiner studies the patient's medical record to decide whether he needed and received skilled nursing care. The examiner may request copies of the patient's monthly bills and look at documented progress notes, especially if the intensity, frequency, and cost of the care increased.

Examiners also check for inconsistencies in documentation, such as a discrepancy between the treatment ordered and the one provided. If the discrepancy isn't explained adequately, the insurer may deny payment.

In addition to barring a facility from reimbursement, faulty documentation can keep patients from getting the care they need. For example, an insurer might deny payment to a home health care agency if the nurse's charting doesn't prove that home visits were necessary. If that happens, home health care may be discontinued prematurely.

PERFORMANCE IMPROVEMENT

Individual states and JCAHO require all health care facilities to regularly monitor, evaluate, and seek ways to improve the quality of care for their patients. In each facility, a committee of physicians, nurses, pharmacists, administrators, and other employees gets together to develop performance improvement measures. Committee members then implement the measures, analyze the improvements, and report their findings to the facility's board of trustees.

Multidisciplinary committee members also develop methods to assess the structure, process, and outcome of patient care. One way to implement these methods is to monitor and evaluate the content of medical records.

What if the care described in a medical record doesn't meet an established standard? Performance improvement committee members must then decide how to correct this problem. They may assign a focus group to investigate ways to do this.

The focus group may recommend changes in the facility's policies, procedures, or documentation forms in an effort to improve patient care. For example, many facilities have been cited in court for lack of documentation when physical restraints were used. As a result, some facilities have developed forms to document restraint orders, which may be used in court as proof that the facility's policy was followed and that restraints were needed.

NURSE PRACTICE ACTS

Nurse practice acts are state laws spelling out what duties nurses can perform in that state. State nurse practice acts are revised frequently; when nurse practice acts change, documentation requirements commonly change as well. With laws and regulations in a constant state of flux, you must be especially meticulous about documenting your care to show compliance with standards.

ACCOUNTABILITY

Accurate nursing documentation is evidence that you acted as required or ordered. Accountability means you comply with the documentation requirements of your health care facility, professional organizations, and state law.

Types of medical records

Medical records — assessment forms, flow sheets, lists to fill out — are kept for every person who steps through the door of a health care facility. How do you deal with all of this?

Many nurses try to create order in medical records by organizing patient data by category, but this emphasizes

TIMESAVER

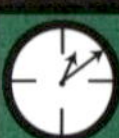

Tips for efficient documentation

When you document, you must record information quickly without sacrificing accuracy. Here are some actions you can take to help you accomplish these two goals:
- Follow the nursing process.
- Use nursing diagnoses.
- Use flow sheets.
- Document at the bedside.
- Individualize your documentation.
- Don't repeat information (this could lead to errors).
- Sign off with your full name and initials.
- Don't document for other caregivers.
- Use computerized documentation.

form instead of content. A medical record isn't just a summary of illness and recovery. It's an insightful record of a patient's care and potential patient care problems.

You can think of the medical record as an ally in your organization efforts. It's a place to organize your thoughts about patient care and to record your actions. Used properly, it can help you save time, identify problem areas, plan better patient care, and avoid litigation. (See *Tips for efficient documentation.*)

Although every medical record provides evidence of the quality of patient care, all records aren't alike. Some are organized by a source-oriented narrative method, some by a problem-oriented method, and others by variations of these two.

SOURCE-ORIENTED NARRATIVE METHOD

With the source-oriented narrative method, caregivers (the source) from each discipline record information in a separate section of the medical record.

This traditional method of documentation has several serious drawbacks: Because charting is done in various parts of the record, information is disjointed, topics aren't always clearly identified, and information is difficult to retrieve. This keeps team members from getting a complete picture of the patient's care and causes breakdowns in communication.

Collaborations among team members who use source-oriented narrative charting are more easily documented if everyone writes on the same progress notes. For example, physicians', nurses', and respiratory therapists' progress notes can be combined into what may be called patient progress notes. These serve as the primary source of reference and communication among health care team members.

PROBLEM-ORIENTED METHOD

A problem-oriented medical record contains baseline data obtained from all departments involved in a patient's care. The problem-oriented charting method is based on the patient's reason for seeking care. Data include:
- the patient's health history, including medical, social, and emotional status
- other initial assessment findings
- diagnostic test results.

CHART QUICK

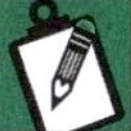

Using problem lists

The chart below shows a nursing problem list for a patient with acute pancreatitis.

#	Date	Problem statement	Initials	Resolved
1	6/4/02	Deficient fluid volume related to vomiting	C.B.	
2	6/4/02	Acute pain related to physiologic factors	C.B.	6/6/02 B.A.
3	6/6/02	Imbalanced nutrition: Less than body requirements related to inability to digest nutrients	B.A.	

The problem-oriented record also contains:

- a problem list
- a care plan for each problem
- progress notes.

The problem list is distilled from baseline data and used to construct a care plan. (See *Using problem lists.*)

The care plan in a problem-oriented medical record addresses each of the patient's problems, which are routinely updated both in the plan and in the progress notes.

OTHER MEDICAL RECORD FORMATS

Some facilities modify the source-oriented or problem-oriented method of documentation to suit their needs. If your facility does this, you're in a position to influence the type and style of documentation you use in medical records.

For example, home health care nurses have created many specialized documentation forms — including an initial assessment form, problem list, day-visit sheet, and discharge summary — to reflect the unique services and the essential quality of care they provide. These forms meet their charting needs while complying with state and federal laws and other regulations.

COMPUTERIZED DOCUMENTATION

Computerized documentation is popular for completing medical records from admission through discharge. Among its benefits, computerized documentation:

- promotes standardization
- eliminates legibility problems that accompany handwritten entries
- may reduce the number of errors
- leads to decreased recording time and costs
- aids communication among team members

Successful automated documentation

To be effective, an automated documentation system must be able to:
- record and send data to the appropriate department
- adapt easily to the health care facility's needs
- display highly selective information on command
- provide easy access and retrieval for all trained personnel.

- allows easier access to medical data for education, research, and performance improvement.

Information filed on computers includes nursing care plans, progress notes, medication records, records of vital signs, intake and output sheets, and patient classifications. Some facilities even have bedside computers for quick data entry and access. (See *Successful automated documentation.*)

The nursing process

The nursing process is a problem-solving approach to nursing care. It's a systematic method for determining the patient's health problems, devising a care plan to address them, implementing the plan, and evaluating the effectiveness of the care.

The nursing process emerged in the 1960s, as team health care came into wider practice and nurses were increasingly called on to define their specific roles. The roots of the nursing process can be traced to World War II, however, when technology, medical advances, and a growing need for nurses began to change the nursing profession.

The nursing process consists of six distinct phases:
- assessment
- nursing diagnosis
- outcome identification
- planning
- implementation
- evaluation.

These six phases are dynamic and flexible and they often overlap. Together, they resemble the steps that many other professions take to identify and correct problems.

ASSESSMENT

The first step in the nursing process—assessment—begins when you first see a patient. Assessment continues throughout the patient's hospitalization as you obtain more information about his changing condition.

During assessment, you collect relevant information from various sources and analyze it to form a complete picture of your patient. As you collect this information, you need to document it accurately for two reasons:
- It will guide you through the rest of the nursing process, helping you formulate nursing diagnoses, expected outcomes, and nursing interventions.
- It will serve as a vital communication tool for other team members and as a baseline for evaluating a patient's progress.

The information that you gather at the first patient contact may indicate that the patient needs a broader or more detailed assessment, such as a nutritional assessment. (See *Assessing nutritional status.*) Further assessment depends on the:

Assessing nutritional status

As part of the admission assessment, the answers to some questions automatically call for another discipline to be consulted. An example is in the nutrition section.

With the following questions, one "no" requires a nutritional consult:

- Do you have sufficient funds to buy food?
- Do you have access to a food market?
- Are you able to shop, cook, and feed yourself?

With the following questions, one "yes" requires a nutritional consult:

- Do you have an illness or condition that made you change the amount or kind of food you eat?
- Do you have any dental or mouth problems that make it difficult for you to chew or swallow food?
- Do you need help in getting to a food market?
- Have you lost or gained 10 lb within the past 6 months without trying?

- patient's diagnosis
- care setting
- patient's consent to treatment
- care the patient is seeking
- patient's response to previous care.

In your initial assessment, take into account the patient's immediate and emerging needs, including not only his physical needs but also his psychological, spiritual, and social concerns. The initial assessment helps you determine what care the patient needs and sets the stage for further assessments. Remember that a patient's family, culture, and religion are important factors in his response to illness and treatment.

Begin your assessment by collecting a health history and conducting a physical examination.

Health history

The health history includes physical, psychological, cultural, spiritual, and psychosocial data. It's the main source of information about the patient's health status and guides the physical examination that follows.

A nursing history differs from a medical history. A medical history guides diagnosis and treatment of illness; a nursing history focuses holistically on the human response to illness.

The nursing history you collect helps you to:

- plan health care
- assess the impact of illness on the patient and family members
- evaluate the patient's health education needs
- initiate discharge planning.

Although nurses conduct health histories in different ways, all interviews must progress in a logical sequence and be an organized record of the patient's response.

Before conducting the health history, consider the patient's ability to participate. If he's sedated, confused, hostile, angry, dyspneic, or in pain, ask only the most essential questions. Then perform an in-depth interview later. In

Obtaining the health history

When you show the patient that you're interested and empathetic, you elicit more accurate and complete answers. Follow these tips to gain an informative health history.

Do

Here are some interviewing do's:

- Use general leads. Broad opening questions encourage the patient to discuss what's important to him.
- Ask open-ended questions. Questions that require more than a yes-or-no answer encourage the patient to express himself.
- Restate information. Summarize the patient's comments and then give him a chance to clarify them.

Don't

These are some things you don't want to do in your interview:

- Don't ask judgmental or threatening questions. Saying "Why did you do that?" or "Explain your behavior" forces the patient to justify his feelings and might alienate him. He might even invent an appropriate answer just to satisfy you.
- Don't ask persistent questions or probe. Make one or two attempts to get information and then back off. Respect the patient's right to privacy.
- Don't offer advice or false reassurance. Giving advice implies that you know what's best for the patient. Instead, encourage him to participate in health care decisions. Saying "You'll be all right" devalues his feelings. But saying "You seem worried" encourages him to speak candidly.

the meantime, ask family members or close friends to provide some information.

Get off on the right foot by finding a quiet, private space where the patient feels as comfortable and relaxed as possible. Ask another nurse to cover your other patients so you won't be interrupted. This reassures the patient that you're interested in what he says and that you'll keep the information confidential. (See *Obtaining the health history.*)

Finding time to conduct a thorough patient history can be difficult. But a few strategies can help you keep interview time to a minimum without sacrificing quality. (See *Making the most of your interview time.*)

Sometimes an interview isn't even necessary — you can simply ask the patient to complete a questionnaire about his past and present health status. Then you can quickly and easily document the patient's health history by reviewing the information on the questionnaire and filing it in the patient's chart. This method is most successful for patients who are to undergo short or elective procedures. The questionnaire can be completed before the patient's admission, which can save you time.

In some acute care settings, modified questionnaires are used to evaluate language and reading problems that the patient may have. The nurse then reviews sections that are completed by the patient.

TIMESAVER

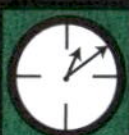

Making the most of your interview time

When you're pressed for time, use the following tips to speed up health history documentation:

- Before the interview, fill in as much information as you can from admission forms, transfer summaries, and the medical history. This avoids duplication of effort. If some information isn't clear, ask the patient for more details. For instance, you might say, "You told Dr. Brown that you sometimes feel like you can't catch your breath. Can you tell me more about when this happens?"
- Check your facility's policy on who may gather assessment data. Maybe you can have an unlicensed nursing assistant or technician collect routine information, such as allergies and past hospitalizations. Remember, though, that reviewing and verifying the information is your responsibility.
- Begin by asking about the patient's reason for seeking medical care. Then, even if the interview is interrupted, you'll still be able to write a care plan.
- Use your facility's nursing assessment documentation form only as a guide to organize information. Ask your patient only pertinent questions from the form.
- Take only brief notes during the interview, so you don't interrupt the flow of conversation. Write detailed notes as soon as possible after the interview. You can always go back to the patient if you need to clarify or verify information.
- Record your findings in concise, specific phrases. Use only approved abbreviations.

Physical examination

The second half of the assessment process involves performing a physical examination. Use the following techniques to conduct the examination:

- inspection
- palpation
- percussion
- auscultation.

The objective data you gather during the physical examination may be used to confirm or rule out health problems that were suggested or suspected during the health history. You rely on these findings in developing a care plan and in your patient teaching. For example, if the patient's blood pressure is high, he may need a sodium-restricted diet and instruction on how to control hypertension.

How detailed should your examination be? That depends on the patient's condition, the clinical setting, and the policies and procedures established by your health care facility. The main components of the physical examination include:

- height
- weight
- vital signs
- review of the major body systems.

(See *Key aspects of the physical assessment*, page 12.)

Key aspects of the physical assessment

During a physical examination, your main task is to record the patient's height, weight, and vital signs and review the major body systems. Here's a typical body system review for an adult patient.

Respiratory system
Note the rate and rhythm of respirations, and auscultate the lung fields. Inspect the lips, mucous membranes, and nail beds. Also inspect sputum, noting color, consistency, and other characteristics.

Cardiovascular system
Note the color and temperature of the extremities, and assess the peripheral pulses. Check for edema and hair loss on the extremities. Inspect the neck veins, and auscultate for heart sounds.

Neurologic system
Assess the patient's level of consciousness, noting his orientation to person, place, and time and his ability to follow commands. Also assess pupillary reactions. Check extremities for movement and sensation.

Eyes, ears, nose, and throat
Assess the patient's ability to see objects with and without corrective lenses. Assess his ability to hear spoken words clearly. Inspect the eyes and ears for discharge and the nasal mucous membranes for dryness, irritation, and blood. Observe the teeth, gums, and condition of the oral mucous membranes, and palpate the lymph nodes in the neck.

GI system
Auscultate for bowel sounds in all quadrants. Note abdominal distention or ascites. Gently palpate the abdomen for tenderness. Assess the condition of the mucous membranes around the anus.

Musculoskeletal system
Assess the range of motion of major joints. Look for swelling at the joints and for contractures, muscle atrophy, or obvious deformity. Assess muscle strength of the trunk and extremities.

Genitourinary and reproductive systems
Note any bladder distention or incontinence. If indicated, inspect the genitalia for rashes, edema, or deformity. (Inspection of the genitalia may be waived at the patient's request or if no dysfunction was reported during the interview.) If indicated, inspect the genitalia for sexual maturity. Also examine the breasts, noting any abnormalities.

Integumentary system
Note any sores, lesions, scars, pressure ulcers, rashes, bruises, or petechiae. Also note the patient's skin turgor.

JCAHO standards

Under JCAHO standards, your initial assessment of the patient should consider:

- physical factors
- psychological and social factors
- environmental factors
- self-care capabilities
- learning needs
- discharge planning needs
- input from the patient's family and friends when appropriate.

PHYSICAL FACTORS

Physical factors include the physical examination findings from your review of the patient's major body systems.

PSYCHOLOGICAL AND SOCIAL FACTORS

The patient's fears, anxieties, and other concerns about hospitalization are psychological and social factors. Find out what support systems the patient has by asking something like, "How does being in the hospital affect your home situation?" A patient who is worried about his family might be less able or willing to comply with treatment.

ENVIRONMENTAL FACTORS

The patient's home environment affects care needs during hospitalization and after discharge. Factors to ask about may include:

- where he lives; whether it's a house or an apartment
- whether he has adequate heat, ventilation, hot water, and bathroom facilities
- how many flights of stairs he has to climb; whether the layout of his home poses any hazards
- whether his home is convenient to stores and medical offices.

In addition, ask if he uses equipment when performing activities of daily living (ADLs) at home that isn't available in the hospital. Tailor your questions to his condition.

SELF-CARE CAPABILITIES

A patient's ability to perform ADLs affects how well he complies with therapy before and after discharge. Assess your patient's ability to eat, wash, dress, use the bathroom, turn in bed, get out of bed, and get around. Some facilities use an ADL checklist to indicate if a patient can perform these tasks independently or if he needs assistance.

LEARNING NEEDS

Deciding early what your patient needs to know about his condition leads to effective patient teaching. During the initial assessment, evaluate your patient's knowledge of the disease process, self-care, diet, medications, lifestyle changes, treatment measures, and limitations caused by the disease or treatment.

One way to evaluate your patient's learning needs is to ask open-ended questions such as "What do you know about the medicine you take?" His response will tell you if he understands and complies with his medication regimen or if he needs more teaching.

You also should assess factors that can hinder learning, which can result from:

- the nature of the patient's illness or injury
- the patient's health beliefs
- the patient's religious beliefs
- the patient's educational level
- sensory deficits such as hearing problems
- a language barrier
- the patient's stress level
- the patient's age
- pain or discomfort.

DISCHARGE PLANNING NEEDS

Discharge planning also should start as soon as possible (in some cases, even before admission), especially if the patient needs help after discharge. Find out where the patient will go after discharge. Is follow-up care accessible? Is there a caregiver who will be available to assist the patient? Are community

CHART QUICK

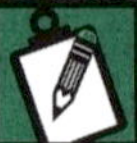

Discharge planning questions

The sample discharge planning form below is one section of the nursing admission assessment form. Use its topics to form your assessment questions.

DISCHARGE PLANNING NEEDS

Living arrangements/caregiver: Sara Smith (patient's daughter)

Type of dwelling: Apartment ___ House ✓ Nursing home ___ Boarding home ___
Other ___

Physical barriers in home: No ___ Yes ✓ Explain: 12 step flight of stairs to bathroom and bedroom

Access to follow-up medical care: Yes ✓ No ___ Explain: ___

Ability to carry out ADLs: Self-care ___ Partial assistance ___ Total assistance ✓

Needs help with: Bathing ✓ Eating ✓ Ambulation ✓
Other ___

Anticipated discharge destination: Home ___ Rehab ___ Nursing home ✓
Skilled nursing facility ___ Boarding home ___ Other ___

resources — such as visiting nurse services and Meals On Wheels — available where he lives? If not, you need time to help the patient make other arrangements. (See *Discharge planning questions.*)

Because inpatient lengths of stay have become shorter and patient care has become increasingly complex, nurses need to prioritize their assessment data. (See *Establishing priorities for patient assessment.*)

INPUT FROM FAMILY AND FRIENDS

Another JCAHO requirement is that you obtain assessment information from the patient's family and friends, when appropriate. When you interview someone other than the patient, be sure to document the nature of the relationship. If the interviewee isn't a family member, ask about and record the length of time the person has known the patient.

NURSING DIAGNOSIS

Your assessment findings form the basis for the next step in the nursing process: the nursing diagnosis. According to the North American Nursing Diagnosis Association, a nursing diagnosis is a clinical judgment about individual, family, or community responses to actual or potential health problems or life processes. Nursing diagnoses are used in selecting nursing interventions to achieve outcomes for which the nurse is accountable.

Each nursing diagnosis describes an actual or potential health problem that a nurse can legally manage. A diagnosis usually has three components:

- the human response or problem — an actual or potential problem that can be affected by nursing care
- related factors — factors that may precede, contribute to, or be associated with the human response
- signs and symptoms — defining characteristics that lead to the diagnosis.

The following nursing diagnosis contains each of these three components: *Ineffective airway clearance related to secretions evidenced by abnormal breath sounds and ineffective cough.*

Familiarity with nursing diagnoses clearly shows how nursing practice and medical practice differ. Although problems are identified in both nursing and medicine, medical and nursing treatment approaches are very different.

The main difference is that physicians and nurse practitioners are licensed to diagnose and treat illnesses, and nurses are licensed to diagnose and treat the patient's response to illness. Nurses also can diagnose the need for patient education, offer comfort and counsel to patients and families, and care for patients until they're physically and emotionally ready to provide self-care.

Whenever you develop nursing diagnoses, you must prioritize them. Then begin your care plan with the highest priority. High-priority nursing diagnoses involve emergency or immediate physical care needs.

Intermediate-priority diagnoses involve nonemergency needs, and low-priority diagnoses involve peripheral needs or those related to enhanced functioning or wellness. Maslow's hierarchy of needs can help you set priorities in your care plan. (See *Maslow's hierarchy of needs,* page 16.)

Establishing priorities for patient assessment

After completion of an initial assessment, the Joint Commission on Accreditation of Healthcare Organizations requires nurses to use the gathered information in prioritizing their care decisions. To systematically set priorities, follow these steps:

- Identify the patient's problems.
- Identify the patient's risk for injury.
- Identify the patient's need for help with self-care, both in the hospital and following discharge.
- Identify the educational needs of the patient and his family members.

OUTCOME IDENTIFICATION

The goal of your nursing care is to help your patient reach his highest functional level with minimal risk and problems. If he can't recover completely, your care should help him cope physically and emotionally with his impaired or declining health.

With this in mind, you should identify realistic, measurable, expected outcomes and corresponding target dates for your patient. Expected outcomes are goals the patient should reach as a result of planned nursing interventions. Sometimes, a nursing diagnosis requires more than one expected outcome.

An outcome can specify an improvement in the patient's ability to function, for example, an increase in the distance

Maslow's hierarchy of needs

To formulate nursing diagnoses, you must know your patient's needs and values. Of course, physiologic needs — represented by the base of the pyramid in the diagram below — must be met first.

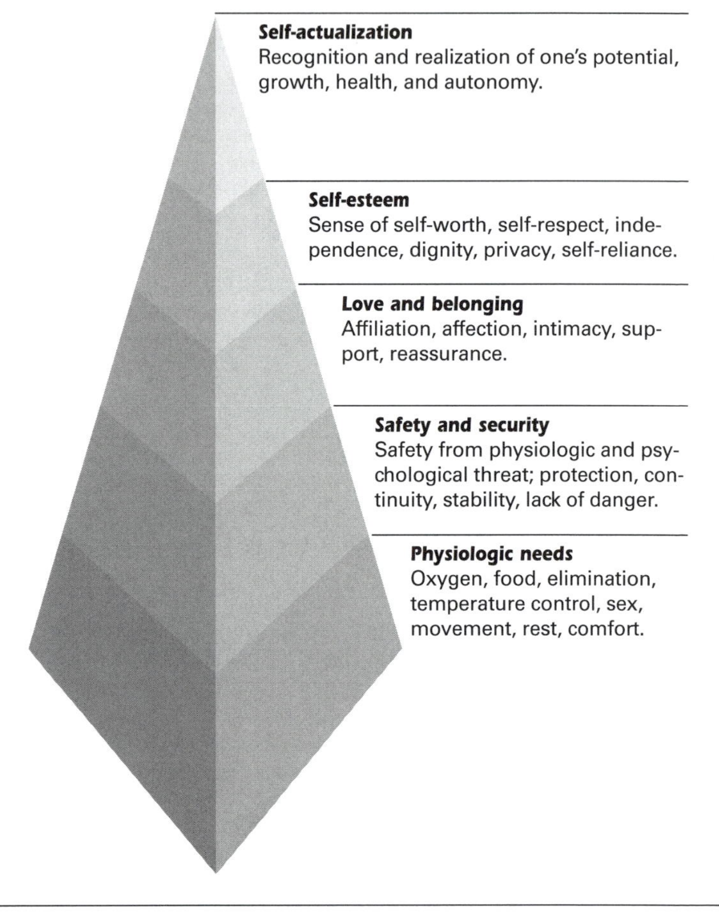

he can walk. Or it can specify the correction of a problem, such as a reduction of pain. In either case, each outcome calls for the maximum realistic improvement for a particular patient.

An outcome statement consists of four parts:

- specific behavior that shows the patient has reached his goal
- criteria for measuring that behavior

Components of an outcome statement

An outcome statement consists of four elements: behavior, measure, condition, and time.

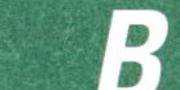

B	M	C	T
Behavior A desired behavior for the patient; must be observable	**Measure** Criteria for measuring the behavior; should specify how much, how long, how far, and so on	**Condition** The conditions under which the behavior should occur	**Time** When the behavior should occur.

As indicated, the two outcome statements below have these four components.

Ambulate	*one flight of stairs*	*unassisted*	*by 5/6/02.*
Demonstrate	*measuring radial pulse*	*before exercising*	*by 5/6/02.*

- conditions under which the behavior should occur
- when the behavior should occur. (See *Components of an outcome statement.*)

Writing outcome statements

Save time when writing outcome statements by choosing your words carefully and being clear and concise. (See *Writing an outcome statement,* page 18.)

Here are some tips for writing efficient outcome statements:

- Avoid unnecessary words. For example, instead of writing *Pt will demonstrate correct wound-care technique by 4/1,* drop the first two words. Everyone knows you're talking about the patient.
- Use accepted abbreviations. Refer to your facility's approved abbreviation list. If it uses relative dates (describes the patient's stay in daylong intervals), use abbreviations, such as *HD 1* for hospital day 1 or *POD 2* for postoperative day 2.
- Make your statements specific. *Understand relaxation techniques* doesn't tell you much; how do you observe a patient's understanding? Instead, *Practice progressive muscle relaxation techniques unassisted for 15 minutes daily by 4/9* tells you exactly what to look for when assessing the patient's progress.
- Focus on the patient. Outcome statements should reflect the patient's behavior, not your intervention. *Medication brings chest pain relief* doesn't say anything about behavior. A correct statement would be *Express relief from chest pain within 1 hour of receiving medication.*

CHECKLIST

Writing an outcome statement

The following tips will help you write clear, precise outcome statements.

❑ When writing expected outcomes in your care plan, always start with a specific action verb that focuses on your patient's behavior. By telling your reader how your patient should look, walk, eat, drink, turn, cough, speak, or stand, for example, you give a clear picture of how to evaluate progress.

❑ Avoid starting expected outcome statements with allow, let, enable, or similar verbs. Such words focus attention on your own and other health team members' behavior — not on the patient's.

❑ With many documentation formats, you won't need to include the phrase *The patient will . . .* with each expected outcome statement. You will, however, have to specify which person the goals refer to when family, friends, or others are directly concerned.

- Let the patient help you. A patient who helps write his outcome statements is more motivated to achieve his goals. His input, along with his family members', can help you set realistic goals.
- Consider medical orders. Don't write outcome statements that ignore or contradict medical orders. For example, before writing *Ambulate 10′ unassisted twice a day by 4/9*, make sure that the medical orders don't call for more restricted activity such as bedrest.
- Adapt the outcome to the circumstances. Consider the patient's coping ability, age, education, cultural influences, family support, living conditions, socioeconomic status, and anticipated length of stay. Also consider the health care setting. For example, *Ambulate outdoors with assistance for 20 minutes t.i.d. by 4/9* is probably unrealistic in a large city hospital.

PLANNING CARE

The fourth step of the nursing process is planning. The nursing care plan is a written plan of action designed to help you deliver quality patient care. It's based on problems identified during the patient's admission interview and consists of:

- nursing diagnoses
- expected outcomes
- nursing interventions.

The care plan becomes a permanent part of the patient's record and is used by all members of the nursing team. Remember, a patient's problems and needs change, so review your care plan often and modify it if necessary.

Writing a care plan involves these three steps:

- assigning priorities to nursing diagnoses
- selecting appropriate nursing interventions to accomplish expected outcomes
- documenting the nursing diagnoses, expected outcomes, nursing interven-

CHECKLIST

Creating a care plan

Use either a traditional or standardized method for recording your care plan. A traditional care plan is written from scratch for each patient. A standardized care plan saves time because it's predetermined, based on the patient's diagnosis.

No matter which method you use, follow these tips to write a plan that's accurate and useful:

❑ Write in ink and sign your name.
❑ Use clear, concise language, not vague terms or generalities.
❑ Use standard abbreviations to avoid confusion.
❑ Review all your assessment data before selecting an approach for each problem. If you can't complete the initial assessment, immediately write "insufficient information" on your records.
❑ Write an expected outcome and a target date for each problem you identify.
❑ Set realistic initial goals.
❑ When writing nursing interventions, consider what to watch for and how often, what nursing measures to take and how to perform them, and what to teach the patient and family before discharge.
❑ Make each nursing intervention specific.
❑ Make sure your interventions match the resources and capabilities of the staff.
❑ Be creative; include a drawing or an innovative procedure if this makes your directions more specific.
❑ Record all of the patient's problems and concerns so they won't be forgotten.
❑ Make sure your plan is implemented correctly.
❑ Evaluate the results of your plan and discontinue nursing diagnoses that have been resolved. Select new approaches, if necessary, for problems that haven't been resolved.

tions, and evaluations. (See *Creating a care plan.*)

IMPLEMENTATION

Next comes selecting interventions and implementing them, the fifth step of the nursing process. Nursing interventions are actions that you and your patient agree will help him reach the expected outcomes. Base these interventions on the second component of your nursing diagnosis, the related factors.

For example, with a nursing diagnosis of *Impaired physical mobility related to arthritic morning stiffness*, select interventions that reduce or eliminate the patient's stiffness such as mild stretching exercises. Write at least one intervention for each outcome statement.

There are several ways to come up with interventions. First, consider interventions that have been successful for you or your patient in the past. For example, if the patient is having trouble sleeping in the hospital and he tells you that a glass of warm milk helps him get to sleep at home, this could work as an intervention for the expected outcome,

Sleep through the night without medication by 4/9.

You also can pick interventions from standardized plans of care, ask other nurses about interventions they've used successfully, or check nursing journals for ideas. If these methods don't work, try brainstorming with other nurses.

Writing interventions

To help you write interventions clearly and correctly, follow these guidelines:

- Clearly state the necessary action. Note how and when to perform the intervention, and include special instructions. *Promote comfort* doesn't say what specific action to take, but *Administer ordered analgesic ½ hour before dressing change* says exactly what to do and when to do it.
- Make interventions fit the patient. Consider the patient's age, condition, developmental level, environment, and values. For instance, if he's a vegetarian, don't write an intervention that requires him to eat lean meat to gain extra protein for healing.
- Keep the patient's safety in mind. Consider the patient's physical and mental limitations. For instance, before teaching a patient how to give himself medication, be sure he's physically able to do it and that he can remember and follow the regimen.
- Follow your facility's rules. For example, if your facility allows only nurses to administer medications, don't write an intervention calling for the patient to *Administer hemorrhoidal suppositories as needed.*
- Consider other health care activities. Adjust your interventions when other activities interfere with them. For example, you might want your patient to get plenty of rest on a day when he has several diagnostic tests scheduled.
- Use available resources. If your patient needs to learn about his cardiac problem, use your facility's education department, literature from the American Heart Association, and local support groups. Write your intervention to reflect the use of these resources.

Documenting interventions

After you have performed an intervention, record the nature of the intervention, the time you performed it, and the patient's response. Also record other interventions that you performed based on his response and the reasons you performed them. This makes your documentation outcome-oriented.

Where you document interventions depends on your facility's policy. You can document them on graphic records, on a patient care flow sheet that integrates all nurses' notes for a 1-day period, on integrated or separate nurses' progress notes, and on other specialized documentation forms such as the medication administration record.

Your facility's policies also dictate the style and format of your documentation. You should record interventions when you give routine care, give emergency care, observe changes in the patient's condition, and administer medications.

EVALUATION

The current emphasis on evaluating your interventions has changed documentation. Traditional documentation didn't always reflect the end results of nursing care. But today, your progress notes must include an evaluation of your patient's progress toward the ex-

Effective evaluation statements

The evaluation statements below clearly describe common outcomes. Note that they include specific details of the care provided and objective evidence of the patient's response to care.

- Response to patient education: *Able to describe the signs and symptoms of hyperglycemia.*
- Response to pain medication within 1 hour of administration: *States leg pain decreased from 9 to 6 (on a scale of 1 to 10) 30 minutes after receiving I.M. meperidine.*
- Tolerance of change or increase in activity: *Able to ambulate to chair with a steady gait, approximately 10', unassisted.*
- Tolerance of treatments: *Unable to tolerate removal of O_2; became dyspneic on room air even at rest.*

pected outcomes you have established in the care plan.

The most commonly used charting method is expected outcomes and evaluation documentation. It focuses on the patient's response to nursing care and helps you provide high quality, cost-effective care. This method is replacing narrative documentation and lengthy, handwritten care plans. (See *Effective evaluation statements.*)

The transition to outcome documentation has been difficult for some nurses. In outcome documentation, the nurse is expected to record nursing judgments, not just nursing interventions. Unfortunately, nurses have traditionally been trained not to make judgments. Today, nurses are being asked to gather and interpret data, refer and prioritize care, and document their findings.

The belief that hands-on care is more important than documentation is one reason nurses often focus more on nursing interventions than on documenting patient responses. Outcomes and evaluation documentation compels nurses to focus on patient responses. And when you evaluate the results of your interventions, you help ensure that your plan is working.

Evaluation of care gives you a chance to:

- determine if your original assessment findings still apply
- uncover complications
- analyze patterns or trends in the patient's care and his response to it
- assess the patient's response to all aspects of his care, including medications, changes in diet or activity, procedures, unusual incidents or problems, and teaching
- determine how closely care conforms to established standards
- measure how well you have cared for the patient
- assess the performance of other members of the health care team
- identify opportunities to improve the quality of your care.

Evaluation itself is an ongoing process that takes place whenever you see your patient. However, how often you're required to make evaluations depends on several factors, including where you work.

If you work in an acute care setting, your facility's policy may require you to review plans of care every 24 hours. But if you work in a long-term care facility, the required interval between evaluations may be up to 30 days. In either case, you still should evaluate and revise the care plan more often if warranted.

Evaluating expected outcomes

Evaluation includes gathering reassessment data, comparing findings with the outcome criteria, determining the extent of outcome achievement (whether the outcome was met, partially met, or not met), writing evaluation statements, and revising the care plan.

Revision starts with determining whether the patient has achieved the outcomes. If they haven't been fully met and you decide that the problem is resolved, the plan can be discontinued. If the problem persists, continue the plan with new target dates until the desired status is achieved. If outcomes are partially met or unmet, identify interfering factors, such as misinterpreted information or a change in the patient's status, and revise the plan accordingly.

Revision to a care plan may involve:

- clarifying or amending the database to reflect new information
- reexamining and correcting nursing diagnoses
- establishing outcome criteria that reflect new information and new or amended nursing strategies
- adding the revised nursing care plan to the original document
- recording the rationale for the revision in the nurses' progress notes.

Documenting evaluation

Evaluation statements should indicate whether expected outcomes were achieved and should list evidence supporting this conclusion. Base these statements on outcome criteria from the care plan, and use action verbs, such as *demonstrate* or *ambulate*.

Include the patient's response to specific treatments, such as medication administration or physical therapy, and describe the condition under which the response occurred or failed to occur. Document patient teaching and palliative or preventive care as well.

After evaluating the outcome, be sure to record it in the patient's chart with clear statements that demonstrate the patient's progress toward meeting the expected outcomes.

Care plans and clinical pathways

The nursing care plan is a vital part of documentation. To the health care team, the nursing care plan is a principal source of information about the patient's problems, needs, and goals. It contains detailed instructions for achieving the goals established for the patient and is used to direct care. It also includes suggestions for solving the patient's problems and dealing with unexpected complications.

There are five aspects to writing the care plan:

- establishing care priorities, based on assessment data
- identifying expected outcomes

- developing nursing interventions to attain these outcomes
- evaluating the patient's responses
- documenting the plan in the format required by your facility.

Until 1991, the care plan wasn't a required part of the patient's permanent record. It was used by the nursing staff and, in some facilities, discarded when the patient was discharged. Now, JCAHO requires that the care plan be permanently integrated into the medical record by written or electronic means.

JCAHO policy changes have also led to greater flexibility when writing plans of care. The commission no longer specifies the format for documenting patient care, so new methods have emerged that can make planning faster and easier.

TYPES OF PLANS

You may write your care plans in one of two styles: traditional or standardized. Whatever approach you use, your care plan should cover all nursing care from admission to discharge. (See *Using care plans,* page 24.)

Traditional care plan

Also called an individually developed care plan, the traditional plan is written from scratch for each patient. After you analyze your assessment data for a patient, you either write the plan by hand or enter it into a computer.

The basic form for the traditional care plan varies, depending on the function of this important document in your facility or department. Most forms have four main columns:

- one for nursing diagnoses
- a second for expected outcomes
- a third for interventions
- a fourth for outcome evaluations.

There may be other columns for the dates when you initiated the plans of care, target dates for expected outcomes, and the dates for review, revisions, and resolutions. Most forms also have a place for you to sign or initial whenever you make an entry or a revision.

What should you include on the forms? This varies, too. Because shorter hospital stays are more common today, in most health care facilities, you're expected to write only short-term outcomes that the patient can reach by the time he's discharged.

However, some facilities — especially long-term care facilities — also want you to chart long-term outcomes for the patient's maximum functioning level. These facilities commonly provide forms with separate spaces for short- and long-term outcomes.

The traditional method has several advantages:

- It provides a personalized plan for each patient.
- The format allows health care team members and the patient to easily visualize the plan.
- Columns for outcome evaluations are clearly delineated.

The main disadvantage of the traditional method is that it's time-consuming to read and write because it requires lengthy documentation.

Standardized care plan

The standardized care plan is commonly used today. A standardized plan eliminates the problems associated with the traditional plan by using preprinted information. This saves documentation time.

CHART QUICK

Using care plans

These samples show how the two types of care plans are organized. Keep in mind that the traditional care plan is written from scratch for each patient, while the standardized care plan needs to be customized for your patient.

TRADITIONAL CARE PLAN

Date	Nursing diagnoses	Expected outcomes	Interventions	Outcome evaluation (initials and date)	Resolution (initials and date)
5/15/02	Decreased cardiac output R/T reduced stroke volume secondary to fluid volume overload.	Lungs clear on auscultation by 5/17/02. BP will return to baseline by 5/17/02.	Monitor for signs and symptoms of hypoxemia, such as dyspnea, confusion, arrhythmias, restlessness, and cyanosis. Ensure adequate oxy-	Lungs clear on auscultation and BP returned to baseline on 5/17/02. (5/17/02, KK)	Resolved (5/17/02, KK)

STANDARDIZED CARE PLAN

Date 4/15/02

Target date 4/16/02

Nursing diagnosis

Decreased cardiac output R/t reduced stroke volume secondary to fluid volume overload

Expected outcomes

Adequate cardiac output (AEB) > 4 L/min
Date met ______ Evaluation ______

Heart rate Apical rate < 90
Date met ______ Evaluation ______

BP 140/80 mm/Hg
Date met ______ Evaluation ______

Pedal pulse palpable and regular
Date met ______ Evaluation ______

Radial pulse palpable and regular

Some standardized plans are classified by medical diagnoses or DRGs; others, by nursing diagnoses. The preprinted information included in a standardized care plan includes interventions for patients with similar diagnoses and, usually, root outcome statements.

Early versions of standardized care plans didn't allow for differences in patients' needs. However, current versions require you to explain how you have individualized the plan for each patient by adding the following information:

- "related to" (R/T) statements and signs and symptoms for a nursing diagnosis. If the form provides a root diagnosis (such as *Acute pain R/T* ________), you might fill in *inflammation, as exhibited by grimacing, expressions of pain.*
- time limits for the outcomes. To a root statement of the goal *Perform postural drainage without assistance*, you might add *for 15 minutes immediately upon awakening in the morning, by 5/12.*
- frequency of interventions. To an intervention, such as *Perform passive range-of-motion exercises*, you might add *twice per day: once in the morning and once in the evening.*
- specific instructions for interventions. For the standard intervention *Elevate patient's head*, you might specify *before sleep, on three pillows.*

When a patient has more than one diagnosis, you have to combine standardized care plans, which can make records long and cumbersome. However, if your facility uses computerized plans, you can extract only the parts you need from each plan, and then combine them to make one manageable plan. Some computer programs provide a checklist of interventions from which you can select to build your own plan.

Although standardized plans usually include only essential information, most provide space for you to write additional nursing diagnoses, expected outcomes, interventions, and outcome evaluations.

Standardized plans of care offer many advantages because they:

- require far less writing than traditional plans
- are more legible
- are easier to duplicate
- make compliance with a facility's policy easier for all members of the health care team, including experts, novices, and ancillary staff
- guide you in creating the plan and allow you the freedom to adapt it to your patient.

This method has one main drawback: If you simply check off items on a list or fill in the blanks, you might not individualize the patient's care or adequately document your findings.

PATIENT-TEACHING PLAN

A patient-teaching plan serves several important functions:

- It pinpoints what the patient needs to learn and how he'll be taught.
- It sets criteria for evaluating how well the patient learns.
- It helps all caregivers coordinate their teaching.
- It serves as legal proof that the patient received appropriate instruction and satisfies the requirements of regulatory agencies such as JCAHO.

To make sure that your teaching plan is as effective as possible, consider carefully what the patient needs to learn, how you'll teach him, and how you'll measure the results. Work closely with the patient, members of his family, and other health care team members to create realistic and attainable goals for your plan. Also provide for follow-up teaching at home, if appropriate.

Be sure to keep your plan flexible. Allow for factors that may interfere with effective teaching, such as a patient's unreceptiveness because of a poor night's sleep or your own daily time constraints.

Parts of the teaching plan

The patient-teaching plan is divided into five sections:

- patient's learning needs
- expected learning outcomes
- teaching content
- teaching methods
- teaching tools.

LEARNING NEEDS

The first step in developing a teaching plan is to identify what your patient needs to learn. Consider what you, the physician, and other health care team members expect him to learn as well as what he expects to learn.

LEARNING OUTCOMES

After identifying the patient's learning needs, you can establish expected learning outcomes, sometimes called learning objectives. Beginning with your assessment findings, list the topics and strategies that the patient needs to learn to reach the maximum level of health and self-care.

Like other patient care outcomes, expected learning outcomes should focus on the patient and be easy to measure. Learning behaviors and the outcomes you develop fall into three categories:

- cognitive — relating to understanding
- affective — dealing with attitudes and feelings
- psychomotor — involving manual skills.

For example, for a patient who is learning to give himself subcutaneous (S.C.) injections, identifying an injection site is a cognitive outcome, coping with the need for injections is an affective outcome, and giving the injection is a psychomotor outcome. (See *Writing clear learning outcomes.*)

To develop precise, measurable outcomes, decide which evaluation techniques best reveal the patient's progress. For cognitive learning, you might use questions and answers; for psychomotor learning, you might use return demonstration.

To measure affective learning — which can be difficult because changes in attitude develop slowly — you can use several evaluation techniques. For example, to determine whether a patient has overcome his anxiety about giving himself an injection, ask him if he still feels anxious. You also can assess his willingness to perform the procedure and observe whether he hesitates or shows other signs of stress while doing it.

Then write the outcome statement based on the selected evaluation technique. For example, if you select return demonstration as your evaluation technique, an appropriate outcome statement might be *Pt demonstrates skill in giving a S.C. injection.*

CONTENT

Next, select what to teach the patient to help him achieve the expected outcomes. Be sure to consult with the patient, family members, and other caregivers in deciding what to teach. Even if the patient is learning self-care, you still should teach a family member how to provide physical and emotional sup-

Writing clear learning outcomes

Learning behaviors fall into three categories: cognitive, affective, and psychomotor. Keeping these categories in mind will help you to write clear, concise learning outcomes. Remember that your outcomes should clarify what you plan to teach, what behavior you expect to see, and what criteria you'll use for evaluating the patient's learning.

Compare the following two sets of learning outcomes:

Poorly phrased learning outcomes	Well-phrased learning outcomes
Cognitive domain	
The patient with heart failure will: • remember his medication schedule. • describe symptoms of heart failure.	The patient with heart failure will: • state when to take each prescribed drug. • recognize when his respiratory rate is increased.
Affective domain	
The patient with heart failure will: • adjust successfully to limitations of disease. • realize the importance of seeing his physician.	The patient with heart failure will: • report feeling comfortable when breathing. • demonstrate willingness to comply with therapy by keeping scheduled follow-up appointments.
Psychomotor domain	
The patient with heart failure will: • take his respiratory rate. • bring in a sputum specimen for laboratory studies.	The patient with heart failure will: • demonstrate diaphragmatic pursed-lip breathing. • demonstrate skill in conserving energy while carrying out activities.

port or how to help the patient remember his care.

When you have decided what to teach, organize your instruction to begin with the simplest concepts and work toward the more complex ones. This is especially helpful when teaching a patient with little education or with learning difficulties.

METHODS

Most of your teaching probably can be done one-on-one. This allows you to learn about your patient, build a relationship with him, and individualize your teaching to his needs.

Many different teaching methods work well along with, or instead of, one-on-one teaching. For instance, try incorporating demonstration, practice, and return demonstration in your teaching plan. Role playing can increase your patient's involvement in the plan, as can case studies, which require him to evaluate how someone else with his disorder responds to different situations.

Other methods include self-monitoring, which requires the patient to assess his situation and to determine which aspects of his environment or behavior need correction. You also can conduct group lectures and discussions if several patients require similar instruction, such as with childbirth or diabetes education.

TOOLS

When choosing tools to help enhance patient education, focus on what will work best for your patient. For instance, if your patient learns best by watching how something is done, try using a videotape of a procedure, a closed-circuit television demonstration, or a slide show.

If the patient learns best by reading, provide written materials, such as brochures and pamphlets. If he prefers a hands-on approach, let him handle the equipment he'll use (for example, syringes, needles, and pumps). If he likes to work independently at his own pace, try an interactive, computerized patient-teaching program. Teaching methods, such as role playing and return demonstration, can optimize your patient teaching.

To get the tools you need, consult the staff-development instructors on your unit, your facility's librarian, or staff specialists. If you can't find what you need, call pharmaceutical and medical supply companies in your community. Also, contact national associations and foundations such as the American Cancer Society. These organizations usually have many patient education materials written for the layperson. They also provide pamphlets and brochures in several languages.

Keep the patient's abilities and limitations in mind as you choose teaching tools. For example, before giving him written materials, such as brochures and pamphlets, make sure that he can read and understand them. Keep in mind that the average adult reads at only a seventh-grade level.

Similarly, make sure you're aware of any language barrier between you and your patient. Use a translator and bilingual aids, such as cards and pamphlets, to overcome this barrier.

Documenting the patient-teaching plan

The patient-teaching plan is a key part of the patient's care plan. By reading it, health care team members can see at a glance what the patient learned and what he still needs to learn. In addition, the health care facility needs the teaching plan to show what quality improvement measures are in progress.

Constructing individual teaching plans requires time and thought. Fortunately, some facilities have patient education departments that develop and implement standard teaching plans for many common disorders.

There are several different forms for documenting your patient-teaching plan. Many of these incorporate the nursing process as it applies to patient education. (See *Using a patient-teaching record,* pages 30 and 31.)

Patient-teaching plans also come in two basic types that are similar to traditional and standardized plans of care. The traditional type begins with the nursing diagnosis statement *Deficient knowledge* and an individualized *related to* statement — for example, *Deficient knowledge related to low sodium diet.* It provides only the format and requires you to come up with the plan.

The standardized type allows you to check off or date steps as you complete them and add or delete information to individualize the plan. It's best suited for patients who need extensive teaching.

Some plans include space for documenting problems that could hinder learning, for comments and evaluations, and for dates and signatures. Or you may need to include this information in your progress notes. No matter which teaching plan you use, this information becomes a permanent part of the patient's medical record.

CLINICAL PATHWAYS

A clinical pathway is an interdisciplinary care plan that describes assessment criteria, interventions, treatments, and outcomes for specific health-related conditions (usually based on a DRG) across a designated time line. A kind of predetermined checklist, it describes the tasks you and the patient need to accomplish. In this way, it's similar to a standardized care plan. However, unlike a care plan, its focus is multidisciplinary, covering all of the patient's problems, not just those identified during a nursing assessment. (See *Following a clinical pathway,* pages 32 to 37.)

Clinical pathways go by many different names: critical pathway, critical path, interdisciplinary plan, anticipated recovery plan, care map, interdisciplinary action plan, and action plan.

Members of the health care team involved in providing care should collaborate to develop each clinical pathway. The goals of the clinical pathway include:

- achieving expected patient and family outcomes
- promoting professional collaborative practice and care
- ensuring continuity of care
- ensuring appropriate use of resources
- reducing cost and length of stay
- establishing a framework for instituting and monitoring continuous quality improvement.

Clinical pathways are most useful in specific types of patient care situations. They work well with high-volume cases (meaning that the facility cares for a lot of patients with this particular problem) and in situations that have relatively predictable outcomes. Complex situations with unpredictable outcomes normally aren't managed with clinical pathways.

A clinical pathway is a permanent part of the medical record. It provides a consistent assessment and documentation tool for third-party payers. It's also used to compare the diagnoses of patients and determine their needs.

Clinical pathways cover the key events that must occur before the patient's target discharge date. These events include:

- consultations

(Text continues on page 36.)

CHART QUICK

Using a patient-teaching record

Use the model patient-teaching form below — for a patient with diabetes mellitus — as a guideline for documenting your teaching sessions clearly and completely.

PATIENT TEACHING
Instructions for patients with diabetes
County Hospital, Waltham, MA

Bernard Miller
7 Main Street
Waltham, MA 04872

Admission date: *6/3/02* Anticipated discharge: *6/8/02*
Diagnosis: *TIA, type 2 DM*

Educational assessment

Comprehension level
Ability to grasp concepts
- ☑ High
- ☐ Average
- ☐ Needs improvement

Comments: ____________

Motivational level
- ☑ Asks questions
- ☐ Eager to learn
- ☐ Anxious
- ☐ Uncooperative
- ☐ Disinterested
- ☐ Denies need to learn

Comments: ____________

Knowledge and skill levels
Understanding of health condition and how to manage it
- ☐ High (>75% working knowledge)
- ☐ Adequate (50% to 75% working knowledge)
- ☑ Needs improvement (25% to 50% working knowledge)
- ☐ Low (<25% working knowledge)

Comments: ____________

Learning barriers
- ☐ Language (specify: foreign, impairment, laryngectomy, other): ____________
- ☐ Vision (specify: blind, legally blind, other): ____________
- ☐ Hearing (impaired, deaf)
- ☐ Memory
  - ☐ Change in long-term memory (specify): ____________
  - ☐ Change in short-term memory (specify): ____________
- ☐ Other (specify): ____________

Instructor's initials: *CW*

Anticipated outcomes

Patient will be prepared to perform self-care at the following level:
- ☑ High (total self-care)
- ☐ Moderate (self-care with minor assistance)
- ☐ Minimal (self-care with more than 50% assistance)

Using a patient-teaching record *(continued)*

Key

P = Patient taught
F = Caregiver or family taught
R = Reinforced
N/A = Not applicable
A = Asked questions
B = Nonattentive, poor concentration
C = Expressed denial, resistance
D = Verbalized recall
E = Demonstrated ability

Date	6/4/02	6/5/02	6/5/02	6/5/02	6/6/02	6/6/02
Time	1900	0800	1330	1830	1000	0800
Assessed educational needs Assessment of patient's (or caregiver's) current knowledge of disease (include medical, family, and social histories)	A/CW					
Assessment of learner's reaction to diagnosis (verbal and nonverbal responses)	A/CW					
General diabetic education goals The patient (or caregiver) will:						
• define diabetes mellitus.	P/A/CW	R/EG	D/ME			D/EG
• state hormone produced in the pancreas.	P/A/CW	R/EG	D/ME			D/EG
• identify three signs and symptoms of diabetes.	P/CW	R/EG	D/ME			D/EG
• discuss risk factors associated with diabetes.	P/CW	R/EG	D/ME			D/EG
• differentiate between type 1 and type 2 diabetes.	P/A/CW	R/EG	D/ME			D/EG
• discuss the importance of careful, regular eye care and examinations.	P/CW	R/EG		D/LT		
• state the importance of oral hygiene.	P/CW	R/EG		D/LT		
Individual goals						
Initial Signature						
CW Carol Witt, RN, BSN						
EG Ellie Grimes, RN, MSN						
ME Marianne Ernst, RN						
LT Lynn Taylor, RN, BSN						

CHART QUICK

Following a clinical pathway

At any point in a treatment course, a glance at the clinical pathway allows you to compare the patient's progress and your performance as a caregiver with care standards. Below is a sample pathway.

Clinical pathway: Colon resection without colostomy

	Patient visit	Presurgery Day 1	O.R. Day	Postop Day 1
Assessments	• History and physical with breast, rectal, and pelvic exam • Nursing assessment	• Nursing admission assessment	• Nursing admission assessment on TBA patients in holding area • Review of systems assessment*	• Review of systems assessment*
Consults	• Social service consult • Physical therapy consult	• Notify referring physician of impending admission		
Labs and diagnostics	• Complete blood count (CBC) • Coagulation profile • ECG • Chest X-ray (CXR) • Chem profile • CT ABD w/wo contrast • CT pelvis • Urinalysis • Barium enema & flex sigmoidoscopy/ colonoscopy • Biopsy report	• Type and screen for patients with hemoglobin (Hb) < 10 g/dl	• Type and screen for patients in holding area with Hb < 10 g/dl	• CBC
Interventions	• Many or all of the above labs/ diagnostics will have already been done • Check all results and fax to the surgeon's office	• Admit by 8 a.m. Check for bowel prep orders • Bowel prep* • Antiembolism stockings	• Shave and prep in O.R. • Nasogastric (NG) tube maint.* • Intake and output (I/O) • VS per routine*	• NG tube maint.* • I/O* • VS per routine* • Catheter care*

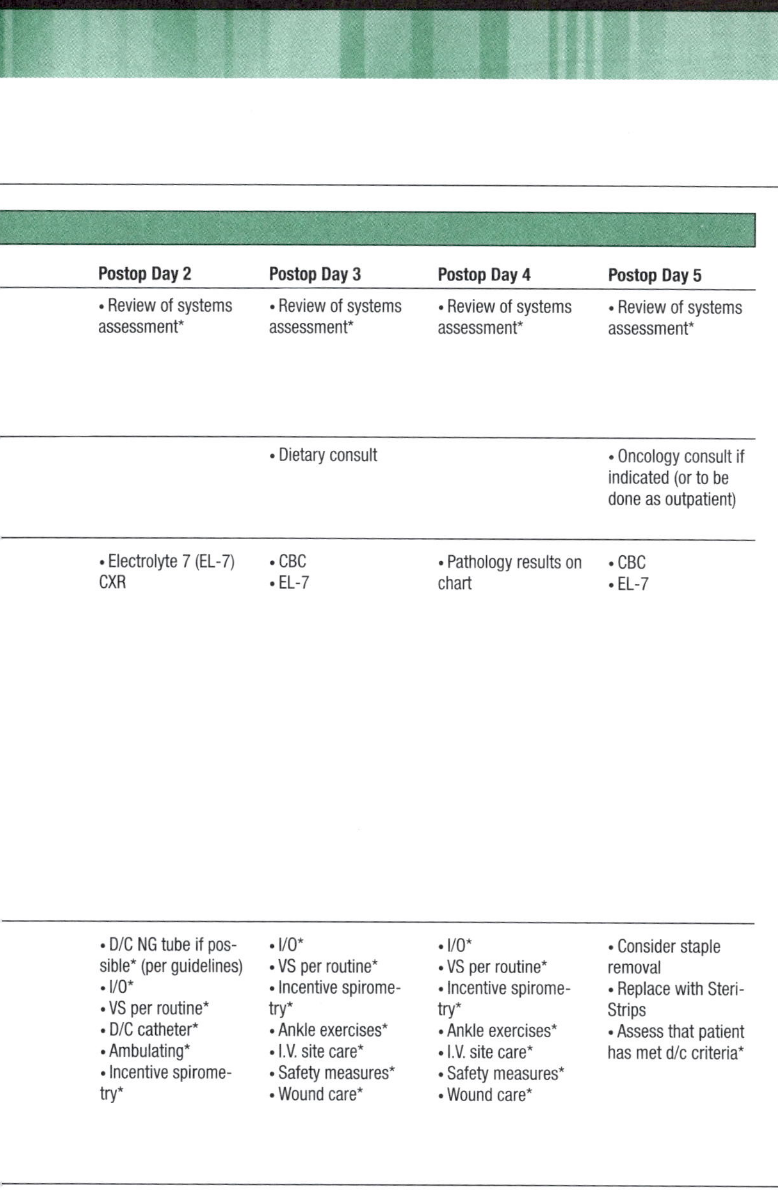

Postop Day 2	Postop Day 3	Postop Day 4	Postop Day 5
• Review of systems assessment*	• Review of systems assessment*	• Review of systems assessment*	• Review of systems assessment*
	• Dietary consult		• Oncology consult if indicated (or to be done as outpatient)
• Electrolyte 7 (EL-7) CXR	• CBC • EL-7	• Pathology results on chart	• CBC • EL-7
• D/C NG tube if possible* (per guidelines) • I/O* • VS per routine* • D/C catheter* • Ambulating* • Incentive spirometry*	• I/O* • VS per routine* • Incentive spirometry* • Ankle exercises* • I.V. site care* • Safety measures* • Wound care*	• I/O* • VS per routine* • Incentive spirometry* • Ankle exercises* • I.V. site care* • Safety measures* • Wound care*	• Consider staple removal • Replace with Steri-Strips • Assess that patient has met d/c criteria*

(continued)

Following a clinical pathway *(continued)*

Clinical pathway: Colon resection without colostomy *(continued)*

	Patient visit	Presurgery Day 1	O.R. Day	Postop Day 1
Interventions *(continued)*		• Incentive spirometry • Ankle exercises* • I.V. access* • Routine VS* • Pneumatic inflation boots	• Catheter care* • Incentive spirometry* • Ankle exercises* • I.V. site care* • Head of bed (HOB) 30°* • Safety measures* • Wound care* • Mouth care*	• Incentive spirometry* • Ankle exercises* • I.V. site care* • HOB 30°* • Safety measures* • Wound care* • Mouth care* • Antiembolism stockings
I.V.s		• I.V. fluids, D_5½ NSS	• I.V. fluids, D_5LR	• I.V. fluids, D_5LR
Medication	• Prescribe – GoLYTELY/ NuLYTELY 10a—2p – Neomycin @ 2p, 3p, and 10p – Erythromycin @ 2p, 3p, and 10p	• Prescribe – GoLYTELY/ NuLYTELY 10a—2p – Neomycin @ 2p, 3p, and 10p – Erythromycin @ 2p, 3p, and 10p	• Preop antibiotics (ABX) in holding area • Postop ABX × 2 doses • PCA (basal rate 0.5 mg) • S.C. heparin	• PCA (basal rate 0.5 mg) • S.C. heparin
Diet/GI	• Clears presurgery day • NPO after midnight	• Clears presurgery day • NPO after midnight	• NPO/NG tube	• NPO/NG tube
Activity			• 4 hours after surgery, ambulate with abdominal binder* • D/C pneumatic inflation boots after patient ambulates	• Ambulate t.i.d. with abdominal binder* • May shower • Physical therapy b.i.d.

Postop Day 2	Postop Day 3	Postop Day 4	Postop Day 5
• Ankle exercises* • I.V. site care* • HOB 30°* • Safety measures* • Wound care* • Mouth care* • Antiembolism stockings	• Antiembolism stockings	• Antiembolism stockings	
• I.V. fluids D_5 ½ NSS+ MVI	• I.V. convert to saline lock	• Saline lock	• D/C saline lock
• PCA (5 mg basal rate)	• D/C PCA • P.O. analgesia • Resume routine home meds	• P.O. analgesia	• P.O. analgesia
• D/C NG tube per guidelines: – (Clamp tube at 8 a.m. if no N/V and residual < 200 ml, D/C tube @ 12 noon)* – (Check with physician first)	• Clears if pt has BM/ flatus • Advance to postop diet if tolerating clears (at least one tray of clears)*	• House	• House
• Ambulate q.i.d. with abdominal binder* • May shower • Physical therapy b.i.d.	• Ambulate at least q.i.d. with abdominal binder* • May shower • Physical therapy b.i.d.	• Ambulate at least q.i.d. with abdominal binder* • May shower • Physical therapy b.i.d.	

(continued)

Following a clinical pathway *(continued)*

Clinical pathway: Colon resection without colostomy *(continued)*

	Patient visit	Presurgery Day 1	O.R. Day	Postop Day 1
Teaching	• Supplement physician's explanation of surgery as necessary*	• Explain all pre- and postop procedures* • Prepare the patient for postop pain and explain that analgesics will be provided*	• Answer all question in clear terms* • Review equipment that patient may experience*	• Reinforce preop teaching*
Key: *NSG activities V = Variance N = No var.	1. V N (N circled) 2. V N 3. V N	1. V N (N circled) 2. V N (N circled) 3. V N (N circled)	1. V N (N circled) 2. V N (N circled) 3. V N (N circled)	1. V N (N circled) 2. V N (N circled) 3. V N (N circled)
Signatures:	1. C. Molloy, RN 2. ________ 3. ________	1. M. Connel, RN 2. C. Roy, RN 3. J. Kane, RN	1. L. Singer, RN 2. J. Smith, RN 3. P. Joseph, RN	1. L. Singer, RN 2. J. Smith, RN 3. P. Joseph, RN

- diagnostic tests
- treatments
- medications
- procedures
- activities
- diet
- patient teaching
- discharge planning
- achievement of anticipated outcomes.

A clinical pathway is usually organized according to categories, such as activity, diet, treatments, medications, patient teaching, and discharge planning. Appropriate categories are determined based on the patient's medical diagnosis. The medical diagnosis also dictates expected length of stay, daily care guidelines, and expected outcomes. Care guidelines are listed under appropriate categories.

The structure of a clinical pathway and the categories it contains vary among facilities. Within a facility, the structure and content of clinical pathways may vary depending on the specific DRG.

Some facilities use nursing diagnoses as the basis for clinical pathways, but this practice is controversial. Critics argue that this format interferes with communication and the coordination of care among non-nursing members of the health care team.

For the most part, clinical pathways are a benefit to nurses for the following reasons:

- They eliminate duplicate charting. The only time you need to write narrative notes is when a standard on the pathway remains unmet or when the patient needs different care than what's

Postop Day 2	Postop Day 3	Postop Day 4	Postop Day 5
• Reinforce preop teaching* • Patient and family education p.r.n.* re: family screening	• Reinforce preop teaching* • Patient and family education p.r.n.* re: family screening • Begin D/C teaching	• Reinforce preop teaching* • Patient and family education p.r.n.* • D/C teaching re: reportable s/s, F/U and wound care*	• Review all D/C instructions and Rx including* follow-up appointments: with surgeon within 3 weeks, with oncologist within 1 month if indicated
1. V (N) 2. V (N) 3. V (N)	1. V (N) 2. V (N) 3. V (N)	1. V (N) 2. V (N) 3. V (N)	1. V (N) 2. V (N) 3. V (N)
1. A. McCarthy, RN 2. R. Mayer, RN 3. P. Drake, RN	1. A. McCarthy, RN 2. R. Mayer, RN 3. P. Drake, RN	1. L. Singer, RN 2. J. Smith, RN 3. P. Joseph, RN	1. L. Singer, RN 2. J. Smith, RN 3. P. Joseph, RN

written on the form. Most pathways provide a place to document alterations in care.

- With standardized orders or protocols, you can advance the patient's activity level, diet, and treatment regimen without waiting for a physician's order. Nurses have more freedom to make care decisions.
- Communication improves between members of the health care team because everyone works from the same plan. That's why problems are called collaborative problems. The goal is for all members of the team to work together to achieve the desired outcome.
- Quality of care improves because of shared accountability for patient outcomes.
- Patient teaching and discharge planning improve. In facilities where clinical pathways are adapted and given to patients, they feel less anxious and are more cooperative because they know what to expect and what's expected of them. Some patients even recover and go home sooner than anticipated.

A significant disadvantage of critical pathways is that they're less effective for patients who have several diagnoses or who have complications. Establishing a time line for these patients is more difficult.

For example, treatment progress is usually predictable for a patient who has a cholecystectomy and is otherwise healthy. But if a patient has diabetes and coronary artery disease, the treatment course is fairly unpredictable, and the care plan is likely to change, resulting in lengthy and fragmented documentation.

Just as you prioritize your nursing diagnoses, you must set priorities for the collaborative problems in the clinical pathway. For example, if your patient needs whirlpool treatments by the physical therapy department and nebulizer treatments from a respiratory therapist, you must coordinate these activities according to the patient's current status and needs.

If everyone on the health care team plans carefully and pays attention to the patient's response to treatments, you should be able to carry out your respective activities for the patient's benefit.

Enhancing your documentation

Documenting like an expert can be simple, but it requires adherence to these seven fundamental rules:

- Document care completely, concisely, and accurately.
- Record observations objectively.
- Document information promptly.
- Write legibly.
- Use approved abbreviations.
- Use the proper technique to correct written errors.
- Sign all documents as required.

Following these rules enhances communication between all members of the health care team and ensures reimbursement for your facility.

DOCUMENTING COMPLETELY, CONCISELY, AND ACCURATELY

Here are a few quick tips for expressing yourself as well as possible:

- Write clear sentences that get right to the point.
- Use simple, precise language.
- Clearly identify the subject of each sentence.
- Don't be afraid to use the word *I*.

Without these tips, a rambling, vague, and ultimately meaningless note might be written such as *Communication with pt's home initiated today to delineate progression of disease process and describe course of action.* That's mind-boggling.

Instead, put the four tips to work for you, and your documentation savvy will show. Here's how this note should be written: *I contacted Andrea Sovak's daughter by phone at 1300 hours; I explained that Mrs. Sovak's respiratory status had worsened and that she would be moved to the ICU for monitoring.* This clearly differentiates your actions from those of the patient, physician, or other staff member.

Because we're taught that nurses don't make diagnoses, many of us qualify our observations with words like *appears* or *apparently*. But using vague language in a patient's chart tells the reader that you aren't sure what you're describing or doing. The right approach is to clearly and succinctly describe what occurred without sounding tentative.

MAINTAINING OBJECTIVITY

Knowing what to document is important as well. Record just the facts — exactly what you see, hear, and do — not your opinions or assumptions. Chart only relevant information relating to patient care and reflecting the nursing process.

Avoid subjective statements such as *Pt's level of cooperation has deterio-*

rated since yesterday. Instead, use the patient's exact words to describe the facts that led you to this conclusion. You might write: *Pt stated, "I don't want to learn how to inject insulin. I tried yesterday, but I'm not going to do it today."*

You may also want to document your subjective conclusion about the patient's condition. This is okay, as long as you also record the objective assessment data that supports it. For example: *Pt sad and tearful with flat affect; states "I miss my family."*

Document only data that you collect or observe yourself or data from a reliable source, such as the patient or another nurse. When you include data reported by someone else, always cite your source. For example, you might write *Nurse Ray found pt attempting to climb OOB; pt was assisted to the bathroom, then back to bedside chair.*

ENSURING TIMELINESS

Timely documentation includes these essentials:

- recording as soon as possible
- noting exact times
- documenting chronologically
- handling late entries correctly.

Record information on the patient's chart as soon as possible after you make an observation or provide care. Information documented immediately is more likely to be accurate and complete. If you don't document until the end of the shift, you might forget important details.

One way to document on time is to keep materials at the patient's bedside. However, this system can threaten confidentiality. (See *Maintaining confidentiality,* page 40.)

If your facility uses computerized documentation, remember that most computerized programs record the date and time that entries are made. Therefore, it's important to specifically state in the body of your note the time that events occurred and the action taken.

Be specific about times in your documentation, especially the exact time of sudden changes in the patient's condition, significant events, and nursing actions. Don't document in blocks of time, such as *5/2/02 0700 to 1500 Pt has NG tube in, vomited once*. This looks vague, implies inattention to the patient, and makes it hard to determine when specific events occurred. Instead, use the exact time, such as *5/2/02 0600 Pt complained of nausea, then vomited 300 ml light brown emesis around NG tube*.

Most facilities require nurses to document in military time, which expresses time as 24 one-hour-long periods per day, rather than two sets of 12 one-hour periods. For example, *0930* refers to 9:30 a.m., and *1950* refers to 7:50 p.m.

Most assessments and observations are useful only as parts of a whole picture. Isolated assessments reveal very little, but in chronological order, they tell the patient's story over time and reveal a pattern of improvement or deterioration.

Documenting in chronological order is easy if you jot down your observations and assessments when they occur. Too often, though, nurses document at the end of a shift, then record groups of assessments that fail to accurately reflect variations in the patient's condition over time. (See *Documenting correctly and chronologically,* page 41.)

If you're using computerized records, know that many software pro-

Maintaining confidentiality

Bedside computers are the ultimate in easy documentation, and bedside flow sheets or progress notes run a close second. However, facility policy must be followed to ensure compliance with confidentiality protocols and regulations.

One solution is to keep confidential records in a locked, fold-down desk outside the patient's room. Having a handy writing surface also makes it easier to document promptly. If your facility doesn't use bedside forms or computers, keep a worksheet or pad in your pocket for note keeping. Just jot down key phrases and times, then transcribe the information onto the chart later.

grams require nurses to answer predetermined questions or fields with multiple-choice answers. Although this approach will capture core data and prompt responses to key issues, it will never replace a patient-specific narrative note. If at all possible, combine a narrative note with the prompted documentation.

Review the documentation entries for the previous 24 to 48 hours. If the record is so generic that you can't identify the patient, then you'll need to incorporate narrative notes in your documentation.

You may occasionally need to add a late entry in certain situations, such as:

- when the chart is unavailable at the time of the event
- when you forgot to document something
- when you need to add important information.

Bear in mind, though, that late entries can look suspicious during a malpractice trial. Find out if your facility has a protocol for late entries. If not, add the entry on the first available line and label it *late entry* to indicate that it's out of sequence. Then record the date and time of the entry as well as the date and time when the entry should have been made.

ENSURING LEGIBILITY

One of the main reasons to document your nursing care is to communicate with other members of the health care team, and legibility is a factor in communication. Trying to decipher sloppy handwriting wastes people's time and puts the patient in jeopardy if critical information is misinterpreted.

Use printing instead of cursive writing because it's usually easier to understand. If you don't have room to document something legibly, leave that section blank, put a bracket around it, and write *See progress notes.* Then record the information fully and legibly in the notes.

Because it's a permanent document, the clinical record should be completed in ink or by computer. Use only black or blue ink. Red and green ink, which are traditionally used on evening and night shifts, don't photocopy clearly. Also, don't use felt-tipped pens on forms with carbon copies because the pens usually don't hold up under the pressure needed to produce copies, and the ink is more likely to bleed through to another page or smear if the paper gets wet.

Notes filled with misspelled words and incorrect grammar create the same

CHART QUICK

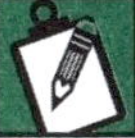

Documenting correctly and chronologically

Here's an example of documentation that's done correctly in chronological order:

5/14/02	0800	Neuro: Pt AAO x 3, follows commands, moves
		all extremities, speech clear and appropriate.
		———— Jane Klass, RN
		CV: Afebrile, skin warm, dry, and intact, palpable
		pulses, no edema. ———— Jane Klass, RN
		Resp: Bilateral breath sounds, no SOB, lungs
		clear, on room air. ———— Jane Klass, RN
		Pt complaining of sudden shortness of breath,
		O_2 2L/minute applied. Stat chest X-ray obtained.
		MD notified. ———— Jane Klass, RN
5/14/02	0920	Lasix 40 mg I.V. provided to pt per Dr. Jones's
		order. ———— Jane Klass, RN
5/14/02	0930	Shortness of breath continues, pulse oximetry
		87%, O_2 increased to 50% face mask. ————
		———— Jane Klass, RN
5/14/02	0935	Pt transferred to ICU, report provided to
		Sally Brown, RN, pt's family notified by MD
		———— Jane Klass, RN

negative impression as illegible handwriting. Try hard to avoid these errors; information can be misrepresented or misconstrued if a error-filled medical record ends up in court. To improve your spelling and grammar, keep both a standard and medical dictionary available in your documentation area. If your computer system includes a spelling or grammar check, use it. And always proofread what you write.

USING ABBREVIATIONS APPROPRIATELY

Standards set by JCAHO and many state regulations stipulate that health care facilities develop a list of approved abbreviations to use during documentation. (See *Abbreviations to avoid,* pages 42 and 43.) Make sure that you know and use your facility's approved abbreviations. When you have doubts about an abbreviation's meaning, spell it out.

Using unapproved or ambiguous abbreviations can endanger a patient. For example, if you use o.d. to mean once a day, another nurse might think you mean oculus dexter (right eye) and instill medication into the patient's eye instead of giving it orally.

CORRECTING ERRORS PROPERLY

When you make a mistake on a chart, correct it immediately by drawing a single line through the entry and writing *mistaken entry* above or beside it, along with the date and time. Then sign your name. Never erase a mistake, cover it with correction fluid, or completely cross it out because this looks as if

Abbreviations to avoid

The Joint Commission on Accreditation of Healthcare Organizations requires every health care facility to develop a list of approved abbreviations for staff use. Certain abbreviations should be avoided because they're easily misunderstood, especially when handwritten. Here's a list of those to avoid.

Abbreviation	Intended meaning	Correction
Apothecaries' symbols		
℥	fluid ounce	Use the metric equivalents.
ʒ	fluid dram	Use the metric equivalents.
♏	minim	Use the metric equivalents.
℈	scruple	Use the metric equivalents.
Dosage directions		
AU	each ear	Write it out.
μg	microgram	Use "mcg."
OD	once daily	Write it out. Don't abbreviate "daily."
OJ	orange juice	Write it out.
TID	three times per day	Write it out.
Per os	orally	Use "P.O.," "by mouth," or "orally."
qn	nightly or at bedtime	Use "h.s." or "nightly."
subq	subcutaneous	Use "S.C." or write it out.
U or u	unit	Write it out.

Abbreviations to avoid *(continued)*

Abbreviation	Intended meaning	Correction
Drug names		
MTX	methotrexate	Use the complete spelling for drug names.
CPZ	prochlorperazine (Compazine)	Use the complete spelling for drug names.
HCl	hydrochloric acid	Use the complete spelling for drug names.
DIG	digoxin	Use the complete spelling for drug names.
MVI	multivitamins without fat-soluble vitamins	Use the complete spelling for drug names.
HCTZ	hydrochlorothiazide	Use the complete spelling for drug names.
ara-a	vidarabine	Use the complete spelling for drug names.

you're trying to hide something. Also, writing *oops* or *sorry*, or drawing a happy or sad face anywhere on a document is unprofessional and inappropriate. (See *Correcting a documentation error,* page 44.)

Changing a record in any way is illegal and constitutes tampering. If the chart ends up in court, the plaintiff's attorney will be looking for red flags that cast doubt on the chart's accuracy. So heed the following list of five "don'ts":

- Don't add information at a later date without indicating that you did so.
- Don't date the entry so that it appears to have been written at an earlier time.
- Don't add inaccurate information.
- Don't omit information.
- Don't destroy records.

If your facility uses computerized records, follow the protocols for the correction of entries made in the chart. Once notes are entered into the computer, they become the permanent record and shouldn't be deleted or edited at a later time without an explanation that's documented, signed, and dated.

SIGNING DOCUMENTS

Sign each entry you make in your progress notes with your first name or initial, last name, and professional licensure, such as *RN* or *LPN*. Your employer may also require that you include your job title. If you find the last entry unsigned, immediately contact the nurse who made the entry and have her sign her name. If you can't locate

CHART QUICK

Correcting a documentation error

When you make a mistake on the clinical record, correct it by drawing a single line through the entry and writing the words mistaken entry above or beside it (don't use an abbreviation like m.e., which could be someone's initials). Follow this with your initials and the date. If appropriate, briefly explain why the correction was necessary.

Make sure that the mistaken entry is still readable. This indicates that you're only trying to correct a mistake, not cover something up.

Correct

Date	Time	Sign entries *Mistaken entry N.C. 6/10/02*
6/10/02	*0900*	~~*Pt. states he is dizzy when changing from sitting*~~
		~~*to standing position*~~ —— *Nancy Cobb, RN*

Incorrect

Date	Time	Sign entries
[illegible]	[illegible]	[illegible] *when changing from sit-*
		[illegible] *position* —— *Nancy Cobb, RN*

her, simply write and sign your own progress notes. The difference in times and handwriting should make it clear which part you've written.

When documentation continues from one page to the next, sign the bottom of the first page. At the top of the next page, write the date, time, and continued from previous page. Make sure each page is stamped or labeled with the patient's identifying information.

Never leave blank spaces on forms. This could imply that you failed to give complete care or to assess the patient completely. If information listed on a form doesn't apply to your patient, write *N/A* (not applicable) in the space. If your documentation doesn't fill the designated space, draw a line through the empty space until you reach your signature at the far right. Don't skip lines; start your progress note on the next available line after the previous entry. Using these tips will prevent anyone from adding a note to yours.

If you need to document the actions of nursing assistants or technicians, write the caregiver's full name — not just his initials. Don't record *Pt assisted to bathroom by nursing assistant.* Include the full name, such as *Pt assist-*

ed to bathroom by Brian Sim, nursing assistant. Many nurses worry about countersigning care that they didn't actually see performed. If this is the case, you may refer to your facility's policy, contact your state board of nursing, or discuss the issue with your nurse-manager. Remember, your signature makes you responsible for everything in the notes.

If your facility uses computerized records, know that most software programs establish an electronic signature based on your personal user password. It's essential to guard your password and not share it with others. This is your legal signature. Always be sure to log off when leaving the computer station. Don't allow anyone else to use the computer with your password logged in. Any entries they make will be stamped with your electronic signature.

Physicians' orders

Almost every treatment you give a patient requires a physician's order, so accurate documentation of these orders is critical. Physicians' orders fall into four categories:

- written orders
- preprinted orders
- verbal orders
- telephone orders.

WRITTEN ORDERS

No matter who transcribes an order — an RN, LPN, or unit secretary — a second person must double-check the transcription for accuracy. An effective method used by many facilities is the "chart check" — rechecking orders from the previous shift once per shift.

Checking for transcription errors at least once every 24 hours is also a good idea. These checks are usually done during the night shift. A line is placed across the order sheet to indicate that all orders above the line have been checked. Then the sheet is signed and dated to verify that the check was done.

When checking a patient's order sheet, make sure that the orders were written for the right patient. An order sheet might be stamped with one patient's identification plate and then inadvertently placed in another patient's chart. Double-checking averts potential mistakes.

If an order is unclear, call the person who wrote the order for clarification. Don't ask other people for their interpretation; they'll only be guessing as well. If a physician is notorious for poor handwriting, ask him to read his orders to you before he leaves the unit.

Some facilities that use a computerized system require the physicians to enter all of their orders into the computer system. This greatly reduces errors because it eliminates transcription.

If you use computerized documentation, be aware that some programs allow you to select more than one patient at a time. Be sure to double-check the patient's name on the computer screen before documenting.

PREPRINTED ORDERS

Many health care facilities use preprinted order forms for specific procedures, such as cardiac catheterization, or admission to certain units such as the coronary care unit. As with other standardized documents, blank spaces are used for information that must be individualized according to the patient's needs.

Using preprinted order forms

When documenting the execution of a prescriber's preprinted order, make sure that you have interpreted and carried out the order correctly. Even though these forms aim to prevent problems (caused by illegible handwriting, for example), they may still be misread. Here are some considerations for using preprinted forms.

Insist on approved forms
Use only preprinted order forms that have your health care facility's approval and the seal of approval of the medical records committee. Most facilities stamp or print an identification number or code on the form. When in doubt, call the medical records department — the prescriber may be using a form he developed or one provided by a drug manufacturer.

Require compliance with policies
To enhance communication and continuity, a preprinted order form needs to comply with facility policies and other regulations. For example, a postoperative preprinted order form shouldn't say "Renew all previous orders" if facility policy requires specific orders. It also shouldn't allow you to select a drug dose from a range ("meperidine 50 to 100 mg I.M. q 4 h," for example) if that's prohibited in your state. Alert your nurse-manager if an order form requires you to perform duties that are outside your scope of practice.

Make sure the form is completed correctly
Many preprinted order forms list more orders than the prescriber wants you to follow, so he'll need to indicate which specific interventions he's ordering. For example, he may check the appropriate orders, put his initials next to them, or cross out the ones he doesn't want.

Ask for clarity and precision
Make sure that the prescriber orders drug doses in the unit of measure in which they're dispensed. For example, make sure that the form uses the metric system instead of the error-prone apothecary system. Report any errors to your nurse-manager.

Promote proper nomenclature
Ask prescribers to use generic drug names, especially when more than one brand of a generic drug is available (for example, "acetaminophen" instead of "Tylenol"). If only one brand of a drug is available, its name can be included in parentheses after the generic name — for example, "dobutamine (Dobutrex)."

Take steps to avoid misinterpretation
Unapproved, potentially dangerous abbreviations and symbols — such as q.d., U, and q.o.d. — don't belong on preprinted order forms. Improper spacing between a drug name and its dosage can also contribute to medication errors. For example, a 20-mg dose of Inderal written as "Inderal20 mg" could be misinterpreted as 120 mg.

Ensure that the copy is readable
If your facility uses a no-carbon-required form, make sure that the bottom copy contains an identical set

Using preprinted order forms *(continued)*

of preprinted orders; this is the copy that goes to the pharmacy. All lines on the bottom copy should also appear on the top copy — extra lines on the pharmacy copy can hide decimal points (making 1.5 look like 15, for example) and the tops of numbers (making 7 look like 1 and 5 look like 3).

If your facility uses these forms, don't assume that they're flawless just because they're preprinted. You may still need to clarify an order by discussing it with the person who gave it. (See *Using preprinted order forms.*)

See the sample preprinted order sheet for an example of appropriate documentation. (See *Preprinted orders,* page 48.)

VERBAL ORDERS

Verbal orders are easy to misinterpret. Errors in understanding or documenting such orders can cause mistakes in patient care and liability problems for you and your facility. So try to take verbal orders only in an emergency when the physician can't immediately attend to the patient. As a rule, do-not-resuscitate and no-code orders should not be taken verbally.

Carefully follow your facility's policy for documenting verbal orders, using a special form if one exists. Here's the usual procedure:

- Record the order on the order sheet as soon as possible. Note the date and time.
- On the first line, write *V.O.* for verbal order. Then write the physician's name and your name as the nurse who received and read the order back.
- Record the order verbatim.
- Sign your name.
- Draw lines through any space between the order and your verification of the order.
- If the order is for a drug, write in ink the drug name, the dosage, the time you administered it, and other information.

Here's an example of documenting a verbal order:

5/16/02 1500 V.O. Dr. Joseph Marks to Mary Jones, RN, Lasix 40 mg I.V. now and daily starting in am.————————————Mary Jones, RN.

Make sure that the physician countersigns the order within the time limit set by your facility. Without this countersignature, you may be held liable for practicing medicine without a license.

TELEPHONE ORDERS

Ideally, you should accept only written orders. However, telephone orders are permissible in the following circumstances:

- The patient needs immediate treatment and the physician isn't available to write an order.
- You're providing care to the patient at home. If so, the orders must be signed by the physician according to state nursing practice regulations. Under Medicare guidelines, verbal orders must be signed within 30 days. Other agencies impose their own, stricter

CHART QUICK

Preprinted orders

The following is an example of a preprinted form for charting a physician's orders. This form specifies the treatment for a patient about to undergo cardiac catheterization.

DISCHARGE PLANNING NEEDS

Allergies: None known

Date/Time	Precardiac catheterization orders:
6/7/02 1330	1. NPO after midnight except for
	medications.
	2. Shave and prep right and left groin areas.
	3. Premedications:
	Benadryl 25 mg } P.O. on call to Cath lab
	Xanax 0.5 mg
	4. Have ECG, PT, PTT, creatinine, Hgb, HCT, and platelet count on
	chart prior to sending the patient to the Cath lab.
6/7/02 1400	5. Have patient void before leaving for the Cath lab.
	———— Mona Jones, MD
	———— Susan Smith, RN

rules. Failure to obtain a signed order could jeopardize reimbursement.

- New information (laboratory data, for example) has become available and the telephone order will enable you to expedite care.

Here's an example of a telephone order:

6/4/02 0900 T.O. Dr. Bartholomew White to Cathy Phillips, RN, Demerol 75 mg and Vistaril 50 mg I.M. now for pain. ————Cathy Phillips, RN.

Telephone orders should be given directly to you; they should never go through a third party. Carefully follow your facility's policy for documenting these orders. Usually, you'll follow this procedure:

- Record the order on the order sheet as soon as possible. First, note the date and time. On the next line, write *T.O.* for *telephone order*. (Don't use *P.O.* for *phone order*—it could be mistaken for *by mouth*.) Then write the physician's name and sign your name.
- Write the order verbatim.
- If you're having trouble understanding the physician, ask another nurse to listen in as the physician gives you the order. Then have her sign the order as well.
- Draw lines through any blank spaces in the order.
- Make sure that the physician countersigns the order within the time limits set by your facility. Without this countersignature, you may be held liable for practicing medicine without a license.
- To save time and avoid errors (and if permitted by your facility's confiden-

WARNING

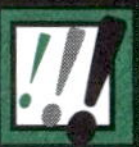

Questioning an order

An order may be correct when issued but incorrect later because of changes in the patient's status. When this occurs, delay the treatment until you have contacted the prescriber and clarified the situation.

Failure to question

In *Poor Sisters of Saint Francis Seraph of the Perpetual Adoration et al. v. Catron* (1982), a hospital was sued for negligence because a nurse failed to question a physician's order regarding an endotracheal tube.

The physician ordered that the tube be left in place for 5 days instead of the standard 2 to 3 days. The nurse knew that 5 days was exceptionally long, but instead of clarifying the physician's order and documenting her actions, she followed the order. As a result, the patient's larynx was irreparably damaged, and the court ruled the hospital negligent.

tiality policy), ask the physician to fax you a copy of the order. Make sure you wait at the fax machine for the transmission, to protect the patient's right to confidentiality.

QUESTIONING ORDERS

Although the unit secretary may transcribe orders, you're ultimately responsible for the transcription's accuracy. Only you have the authority and the knowledge to question the validity of orders and to spot errors. This is why a chart check is so important.

What if an order seems vague or even wrong? Refuse to carry it out until you talk to the physician. (See *Questioning an order.*) Your facility should have a written procedure for clarifying orders. If it doesn't, take these steps:

- Contact the prescriber for clarification.
- Document that you did this.
- Document whether you carried out the order.
- If you refuse to carry out an order, document your refusal, including the reasons why you refused and your communications with the physician. Inform your immediate supervisor.
- Ask your nursing administrator for a step-by-step policy to follow so you'll know what to do if the situation recurs.

Sometimes an order is correct when it's given, then it becomes incorrect later because the patient's status changes. When this occurs, delay the treatment until you have contacted the physician for clarification.

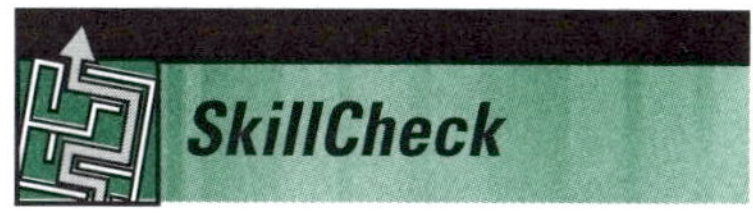

1. If you make a documentation error in the clinical record, you should:

a. use correction fluid to completely cover the error, then sign and date it.

b. erase the error completely, then

initial and date it.

c. draw a single line through the error, write *mistaken entry* above or beside it, and initial and date it.

d. use ink to completely cross out the error, then sign and date it.

Answer: c. An error should never be erased, completely crossed out, or covered with correction fluid; it looks as if you're trying to hide something.

2. Discharge planning should begin:

a. before or on the day of admission.

b. on the second day after admission.

c. several days before discharge.

d. the day of discharge.

Answer: a. Discharge planning should start as soon as possible (in some cases, even before admission), especially if the patient will need help after discharge.

3. Documenting completely, concisely, and accurately can be done by doing all of the following, except:

a. writing clear sentences that get right to the point.

b. not using long words when short ones will do.

c. clearly identifying the subject of each sentence.

d. never using the word *I.*

Answer: d. Don't be afraid to use the word *I;* it clearly differentiates your actions from those of the patient, physician, or other staff member.

4. Which of the following is the best outcome statement?

a. *Will ambulate by 6/8/02.*

b. *Understands the need to take deep breaths.*

c. *Will be free from pain by 6/8/02.*

d. *Demonstrates using incentive spirometer 3x's daily, unassisted, by 6/8/02.*

Answer: d. Remember that an outcome statement should consist of these four elements: behavior, measure, condition, and time.

5. The nursing health history is most accurately described as:

a. a tool to guide diagnosis and treatment of the illness.

b. a follow-up to the medical history.

c. an interview that focuses holistically on the human response to illness.

d. a summary of the patient's current problem.

Answer: c. Focusing holistically on the human response to illness is how the nursing health history differs from a medical health history, which focuses on diagnosis and treatment.

2 Legal aspects of documentation

As your professional responsibility grows, so does your legal accountability. Complete, accurate documentation proves that you're giving quality care and meeting the standards set by the nursing profession, your health care facility, and the law. It's your best protection if you're named in a malpractice lawsuit. (See *The medical record in court,* page 52.)

Faulty documentation is a pivotal issue in many malpractice cases. Medical records are reviewed by health care experts and can be presented in court case trials. Think of the medical record as a communication tool and document accordingly. Focus on the facts, be objective, and document chronologically.

Legal standards

What and how you document on the medical record is controlled by:

- your state's nurse practice acts
- American Nurses Association (ANA) credentialing committee certification requirements
- malpractice litigation
- your facility's policies and procedures.

NURSE PRACTICE ACTS

Nurse practice acts are state laws that designate what a nurse can do in that state. Today, nurses are considered managers of care as well as practitioners; states revise their laws and documentation requirements to keep up with changes like this in the nursing profession.

The range of a nurse's legal responsibilities may vary from state to state—perhaps only to a small degree in certain cases. However, when licensed in more than one state, you must take care to follow precisely the specific guidelines of the state you're practicing in at the time. Always be familiar with your scope of practice. You'll be held liable if found practicing outside of your designated scope of practice.

ANA CREDENTIALING

What you write in a medical record shouldn't be dictated by the courts; it should be guided by the nursing profession's own standards. Documentation that meets these standards describes the patient's status, medical treatment, and nursing care. The ANA sets standards for most nursing specialties. It says that documentation must be:

- systematic
- continuous
- accessible
- communicated
- recorded
- readily available to all members of the health care team.

WARNING

The medical record in court

The outcome of every malpractice trial comes down to one question: Whom will the jury believe? The answer depends on the credibility of the evidence. Jurors usually view the medical record as the best evidence of what really happened. It's often the hinge on which the verdict swings.

A general overview

Briefly, this is what happens in court: The plaintiff's (patient's) attorney presents evidence showing that the patient was harmed because care provided by the defendant (in this case, the nurse) failed to meet accepted standards. The nurse's attorney presents evidence showing that his client provided a standard of care that would be used by other nurses given the same circumstances.

If the nurse wasn't negligent, the medical record will provide evidence of quality care. But if she was negligent and truthfully documented her care, the medical record is the plaintiff's best evidence. The jury will almost certainly rule in favor of the patient. Don't believe the myth that all cases settle out of court. Some do, but you don't want to be the exception.

While documentation goals haven't changed much over the years, documentation methods have. Nurses now use flow sheets, graphic records, and checklists in place of long narrative notes. In malpractice cases, the documentation method used isn't important, as long as it's used consistently and provides comprehensive, factual information that's relevant to the patient's care.

MALPRACTICE LITIGATION

When documenting, your main goal is to convey information. However, keep the legal implications in the back of your mind. If the care you provide and your documentation are both top-notch, the records may be used to refute a plaintiff's accusation of nursing malpractice.

A malpractice verdict depends on these three factors:

- breach of duty
- damage
- causation.

The courts have ruled that your duty is to provide an appropriate standard of care when a nurse-patient relationship is established—even if the relationship takes place over the phone. Breach of duty means that your care didn't meet that standard.

Proving that a nurse was guilty of breach of duty is difficult because nursing duties overlap with those of other health care providers. The court will ask: "How would a reasonable, prudent nurse with comparable training and experience have acted in the same or a similar circumstance?"

When the plaintiff establishes a breach of duty, he must then prove that the breach caused the patient's injury (damage and causation).

FACILITY POLICIES AND PROCEDURES

How you document is also controlled by the policies and procedures in your facility's employee and nursing manuals. Straying from these rules suggests that you failed to meet the facility's standards of care.

While the courts have yet to decide whether these policies actually establish a legal standard of care, there are legal standards in place. In each nursing malpractice case, the courts compare a nurse's actions with regularly updated, national minimum standards established by professional organizations and accrediting bodies, such as the Joint Commission on Accreditation of Healthcare Organizations.

According to insurance company data, lawsuits naming nurses as defendants are increasing. Why? A nurse's expanding role and the breakdown of the nurse-patient relationship due to shorter hospital stays are two reasons.

Developing a rapport with your patients, even on a short-term basis, can help decrease errors and foster a nurse-patient relationship; both of which help prevent lawsuits. Patients who feel their nurse attempted to do all in her power to provide care — often despite the probability of short staffing — typically don't sue the nurse. However, they may sue the facility as the responsible party.

Guidelines for documentation

In the world of nursing and malpractice, a defensive attitude has become necessary — that is, document factually but defensively as well. This involves knowing:

- how to document
- what to document
- when to document
- who should document.

HOW TO DOCUMENT

A skilled nurse documents with possible litigation in mind and knows that how she documents is just as important as what she documents.

Document the facts

Record only what you see, hear, smell, feel, measure, and count — not what you suppose, infer, conclude, or assume. For example, if a patient pulled out his I.V. line, but you didn't witness it, write: *Found pt, arm board, and bed linens covered with blood. I.V. line and venipuncture device were untaped and hanging free.* If the patient says he pulled out his I.V. line, record that using quotations and the patient's exact words.

Don't document your opinions. If the chart is used as evidence in court, the plaintiff's attorney might attack your credibility and the medical record's reliability.

Avoid labeling

Objectively describe the patient's behavior instead of subjectively labeling it. Expressions like *appears spaced out, flying high, exhibiting bizarre behavior,* or *using obscenities* mean different things to different people. Could you define these terms in court? Documenting objectively will increase your credibility with the jury.

Be specific

Your goal is to present the facts clearly and concisely. To do so, use only approved abbreviations and express your observations in quantifiable terms.

For example, writing *output adequate* isn't as helpful as writing *output 1,200 ml*. And *Pt appears to be in pain* is vague compared to *Pt requested pain medication after complaining of lower back pain radiating to his right leg with a VAS (Visual analogue scale) 7/10*. Also, avoid catch-all phrases such as *Pt comfortable*. Instead, describe how you know this. For instance, is the patient resting, reading, or sleeping?

Use neutral language

Don't use inappropriate comments or language in your notes. This is unprofessional and can cause legal problems.

In one case, an elderly patient developed pressure ulcers, and his family complained that he wasn't receiving adequate care. The patient later died, probably of natural causes. Because family members were dissatisfied with the patient's care, they sued. The insurance company questioned the abbreviation *PBBB* in the chart, which the physician had written under prognosis. After learning that this stood for "pine box by bedside," the family was awarded a significant sum.

Eliminate bias

Don't use language that suggests a negative attitude toward the patient. Examples include *obstinate*, *drunk*, *obnoxious*, *bizarre*, or *abusive*. The same goes for what you say out loud and then document. Disparaging remarks, accusations, arguments, or name calling could lead to a defamation of character or libel suit. In court, the plaintiff's attorney might say, "This nurse called my client 'rude, difficult, and uncooperative.' It's right here in her own handwriting! No wonder she didn't take good care of him—she didn't like him." Remember, the patient has a legal right to see his chart. If he spots a derogatory reference, he'll be hurt, angry, and more likely to sue.

If a patient is difficult or uncooperative, document the behavior objectively and let the jurors draw their own conclusions. (See *Documenting difficult situations*.)

Keep the record intact

Be sure to keep the patient's chart complete. Discarding pages, even for innocent reasons, raises doubt in an attorney's mind.

Let's say that you spill coffee on a page and blur several entries. Don't discard the original! Copy it and put the copy and the original in the chart. Then cross-reference the pages by writing, *Recopied from page___* on the copy and *Recopied on page___* on the original.

WHAT TO DOCUMENT

Caring for patients seems more important than documenting every detail, doesn't it? However, legally speaking, an incomplete chart reflects incomplete nursing care. Deleting details is such a serious and common documentation error that malpractice attorneys have coined the expression "Not charted, not done."

This doesn't mean that you have to document everything. Some information, like staffing shortages and staff conflicts, is definitely off limits. (See *Charting don'ts,* pages 56 and 57.)

CHART QUICK

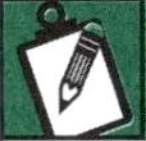

Documenting difficult situations

The note below describes a difficult situation dispassionately, while still getting the point across.

6/17/02	1300	I attempted to perform the daily abdominal
		dressing change, pt stated, "This doesn't need
		to be done every day. It doesn't hurt and I
		don't want you to touch it. Leave me alone." I
		explained the importance of monitoring and
		cleaning the incision, and offered an analgesic
		to be given 20 minutes before dressing would
		be changed. Pt became agitated and still
		refused. Dr. Humbert notified that incisional
		site was not assessed nor was dressing changed,
		and that pt is agitated. ——— Mary Marley, RN

Document significant situations

Learn to recognize legally dangerous situations as you give patient care. Assess each critical or out of the ordinary situation and decide whether your actions might be significant in court. If they could be, document them as well as every other detail of the situation. (See *A case of negligence,* page 58, and *Documenting atypical situations,* page 59.)

Document complete assessment data

Failing to perform and document a complete physical assessment is a key factor in many malpractice suits. During your initial assessment, focus on the patient's reason for seeking care, and then follow up on all other problems he mentions. Be sure to document everything you do and why.

After completing the initial assessment, write a well-constructed care plan. This gives you a clear approach to the patient's problems and helps defend your care if you're sued.

Phrase each problem statement clearly, and modify them as you gather new assessment data. State the care plan for solving each problem; then identify the actions you intend to take.

Document discharge instructions

Because of insurance constraints, facilities are discharging patients earlier than they used to. This means that patients and family members are changing dressings, assessing wounds, and tackling other tasks that nurses traditionally performed.

Patient and family teaching are your responsibility. If a patient receives inadequate or incorrect instructions and an injury results, you could be held liable.

Many facilities give patients printed instruction sheets that describe treatments and home care procedures. In court, these materials may be used as evidence that instruction took place. To

Charting don'ts

Negative language and inappropriate information don't belong in a medical record and may be used against you in a lawsuit. The charting mistakes below are legal land mines. Avoid them.

- **Don't record staffing problems**

True, staff shortages may affect patient care or contribute to an incident. But don't mention this in a patient's chart; it can be used as legal ammunition against you if the chart lands in court. Instead, write a confidential memo to your nurse-manager, and review your facility's policy and procedure manuals to see how you're expected to handle this situation. Remember, the medical record isn't a forum for recording health care issues.

- **Don't record staff conflicts**

Don't document:

- disputes with other nurses (including criticisms of their care)
- questions about a physician's treatment
- a colleague's rude or abusive behavior.

Personality clashes aren't legitimate patient care concerns. In the event of a lawsuit, the plaintiff's attorney will exploit conflicts among codefendants.

Instead of documenting these problems, talk with your nurse-manager, or consult with the physician directly if an order puzzles you. If another nurse writes personal accusations or charges of incompetence in a chart, talk to her about the implications of doing this. Keep in mind that you're responsible for your actions and behavior.

- **Don't mention incident reports**

Incident reports are confidential and filed separately from the patient's chart. Document only the facts of an incident in the chart, and never write "incident report" or indicate that you filed one.

For example, write: *Found pt lying on the floor at 1250 hours. Vital signs: BP 110/70, P 82, R 20, T 98.6. No visible bleeding or trauma. AAOx3, PERLA, + ROM to all extremities. Pt returned to bed with all side rails up and bed in low position. Pt stated, "I must have been sleepwalking." Notified Dr. Gary Dietrich at 1253 hours, and he saw pt at 1300 hours, no orders written.*

- **Don't use words associated with errors**

Terms like "by mistake," "accidentally," "somehow," "unintentionally," "miscalculated," and "confusing" are bonus words to the plaintiff's attorney. Steer clear of words that suggest an error was made or a patient's safety was jeopardized. Let the facts speak for themselves.

For example, suppose you gave a patient 100 mg of Demerol instead of 50 mg. Here's how to chart this without calling undue attention to it: *Pt was given Demerol 100 mg I.M. at 1300 hours for abdominal pain VAS 7/10. Dr. Smith notified, no orders written. Pt's vital signs remained stable.*

Charting don'ts *(continued)*

- **Don't name a second patient**
Naming a second patient in a patient's chart violates confidentiality. Instead, write roommate, the patient's initials, or his room and bed number.
- **Don't document casual conversations with colleagues**
Telling your nurse-manager in the elevator or restroom about a patient's deteriorating condition doesn't qualify as informing her. She's likely to forget the details or may not even realize you expect her to intervene. Before notifying someone, clearly state why you're notifying the person so she can focus on the facts and take appropriate action. Otherwise, you can't document that you informed her.

support testimony, they should be tailored to each patient's specific needs and contain any verbal or written instructions you provided. Documentation of referrals to home health care agencies or other community providers is another essential component of discharge planning.

WHEN TO DOCUMENT

Finding time to document can be hard during a busy shift. But the timeliness of entries is a major issue in malpractice suits.

Document nursing care when you perform it or shortly afterward. Never document ahead of time—your notes will be inaccurate and you'll leave out information about the patient's response to treatment. Even if you did what you recorded, an attorney might ask, "Do you occasionally document something before doing it?" If you answer yes, the jury won't see the chart as a reliable indicator of what you actually did, which forfeits your credibility.

WHO SHOULD DOCUMENT

State nurse practice acts have strict rules about who can document. Breaking these rules can cause you to have your nursing license suspended.

No matter how busy you are, never ask another nurse to complete your documentation (and never complete another nurse's documentation). Doing so is a dangerous practice that may be specifically prohibited by your state's nurse practice act. If the other nurse makes an error or misinterprets information, the patient can be harmed. Then, if he sues you for negligence, both you and your facility will be held accountable because delegated documentation doesn't meet nursing standards.

Delegating documentation has another consequence: It destroys the credibility and value of the medical record in the facility and in court. Judges give little if any weight to medical records containing secondhand observations or hearsay evidence.

WARNING

A case of negligence

Here's a fictional case that exemplifies how negligence may be interpreted in court.

Seventeen-year-old Tommy York was partially paralyzed and severely brain damaged after an accident. He was admitted to the hospital for an intensive rehabilitation program.

Soon afterward, his parents told the nurse that a support from the right side of his wheelchair was missing and that they saw scratches on his right arm. Although the nurse also noticed this, she didn't record it.

Failure to document

Later, the patient's hip became red, swollen, and increasingly painful. His mother also reported these symptoms to the nurse, who again failed to record them in the medical record.

When the patient was finally diagnosed with a broken hip, his parents sued. The court ruled the hospital negligent and awarded the plaintiff $250,000.

A matter of duty

Inadequate observation of patients that leads to misdiagnosis or injury is a common cause of lawsuits involving nurses. Most of these lawsuits involve issues of negligence — failure to exercise the degree of care that a person of ordinary prudence would exercise under the same circumstances. A claim of negligence requires that there be a duty owed by one person to another, that the duty be breached, and that injury result.

Malpractice is a more restricted type of negligence, defined as a violation of professional duty to act with reasonable care and in good faith. Several states have begun to recognize nursing negligence as a form of malpractice.

Avoid negligence cases by documenting all unusual patient events.

Risk management and documentation

A health care facility's reputation for safe, reliable, effective service is its main defense against liability claims. Well-coordinated risk management and quality assurance programs show the public that the facility is being managed in a legally responsible manner. If complaints arise, a good program ensures that they're handled promptly to contain the damage and minimize liability claims. (See *Understanding risk management and performance improvement*, page 60.)

Sometimes documentation reveals potential problems within a health care facility. For example, a certain procedure may repeatedly lead to patient injury or another type of accident. Risk management programs help reduce injuries and accidents and thereby minimize financial loss.

In the past, the focus of risk management and performance improvement programs was to maintain and improve facilities and equipment and ensure employee, visitor, and patient safety. But today, the focus is on identifying, evaluating, and reducing patient

CHART QUICK

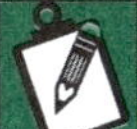

Documenting atypical situations

This note shows the right way to document information that's out of the ordinary.

6/18/02	1900	Furosemide 40 mg P.O. not given because pt now
		NPO for impending upper GI series. Dr. Wenger
		notified that furosemide was not given. Dr. Wenger
		gave order for furosemide 20 mg I.V. Administered
		at 1915. ———— Charles Cashman, RN

injury in all areas of a facility and by all its personnel.

PREVENTING ADVERSE EVENTS

Risk management has three main goals:

- decreasing the number of claims by promptly identifying and following up on adverse events (early warning systems)
- reducing the frequency of preventable injuries and accidents leading to lawsuits by maintaining or improving the quality of care
- controlling costs related to claims by pinpointing trouble spots early and working with the patient and his family.

Early warning systems

Early warning systems can pinpoint much useful information, but to be effective they need:

- a strong organizational structure
- cooperation between risk management and quality assurance departments
- the commitment of all staff members to report adverse events to the appropriate clinical chairperson, so he can study the medical records more closely or talk to the staff member involved and recommend remedial education, monitoring, or restricted privileges
- the commitment of key staff members — such as nurses, doctors, administrators, and chiefs of high-risk services — to analyze the information
- the commitment of all staff members to be compliant with policies and procedures to maintain and maximize quality patient care.

The most commonly used early warning systems are occurrence reporting and occurrence screening.

OCCURRENCE REPORTING

An occurrence or incident report refers to the documentation of events that are inconsistent with a health care facility's ordinary routine, regardless of whether injury occurs. Physicians, nurses, or other staff are responsible for reporting such events when they're observed or shortly afterward. Examples include the unplanned return of a patient to the operating room or a medication error.

Understanding risk management and performance improvement

Do the terms *risk management* and *performance improvement* confuse you? Here's how to tell them apart: Risk management focuses on patients' and family members' perceptions of the care provided, whereas peformance improvement focuses on the role of the health care provider.

Many facilities combine these two programs in their educational efforts. They place a high priority on teaching new medical residents and nurses about malpractice claims, staff members' reporting obligations, proper informational and reporting channels, and principles of risk management and quality assurance.

OCCURRENCE SCREENING

Occurrence screening involves reviewing medical records to find adverse events. Both general indicators of adverse events (such as a nosocomial infection or medication error) and more specific indicators (such as an incorrect sponge count during surgery) are considered.

MANAGING INCIDENTS

Despite risk management programs, adverse events still occur. Health care facilities rely on the following sources to identify dangerous situations or trends:

- Incident reports, also called occurrence reports, are also a primary source of information for attorneys. They use the reports when researching potential lawsuits and in court as evidence.
- Nurses are usually the first ones to recognize potential problems because they spend so much time with patients and families. They know which patients are dissatisfied with their care and which ones have complications that may lead to injuries.
- Patient-representatives keep files of patient complaints, identify litigious patients, and maintain contact with the patient and his family after an incident has occurred.
- The business office and medical records department may be alerted to potential lawsuits when a patient threatens to sue after he receives his bill or when a patient or an attorney requests a copy of the medical record.
- Other sources — for example, the engineering department — has information on the safety of the hospital environment; purchasing, biomedical engineering, and the pharmacy can report on the safety and adequacy of products and equipment; and social workers, hospital clergy, volunteers, and patient escorts often know about highly dissatisfied patients. Remember: Whenever you get a report from one of these sources, document it thoroughly in the patient's medical record and fill out an incident report.

When the risk manager learns of a potential or actual lawsuit, he notifies the medical records department and the facility's insurance company. The medical records department makes copies of the patient's chart and files the original in a safe place to prevent tampering.

A claim notice should also trigger a quality assurance peer review of the medical record. This review measures the health care provider's conduct against the professional standards of conduct for the particular situation. This information is used by the risk manager to investigate the claim's merit and the facility's responsibility in that situation. The standard required for a successful defense isn't always as high as the facility's optimal standard.

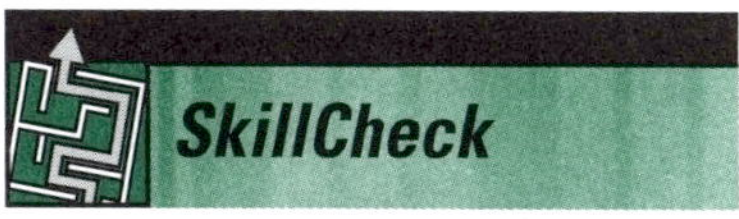

1. Accurate, complete documentation in the medical record benefits the nurse in all of the following ways, except:

a. it proves that you're giving quality care.
b. it proves that you're meeting the care standards set by the nursing profession, your health care facility, and the law.
c. it isn't admissible in court.
d. it's a reliable indicator of the care you performed.

Answer: c. The medical record is admissible in court, and your accurate and complete documentation will be your best protection if you're named in a lawsuit.

2. Who should document the nursing care that you perform?

a. Your nurse-manager
b. Another nurse designated by you
c. The unit secretary
d. You, and only you

Answer: d. Delegated nursing documentation may be prohibited by some nurse practice acts and may not be viewed as credible evidence in court because it would contain secondhand observations or hearsay.

3. It's best to document your nursing care:

a. at the end of your shift.
b, when you perform it or shortly after.
c. ahead of time.
d. the next day.

Answer: b. To preserve the credibility of your documentation, it should be done as soon as possible after you perform care; it's the most reliable indicator of what you actually did.

4. If you're named as a defendant in a malpractice suit, your actions will be compared with those of:

a. your nurse-manager.
b. a physician.
c. the patient's expectations.
d. a reasonable, prudent nurse with comparable training and experience.

Answer: d. Your actions would be compared with those of a nurse, who meets the above qualifications, in the same or a similar circumstance.

5. All of the following elements are necessary to make a claim of malpractice, except:

a. an uncooperative patient.
b. a duty owed by one person to another.
c. a breech of duty.
d. a resulting injury.

Answer: a. Regardless of the patient involved, a negligence claim can be made when there is a duty owed, a breech of that duty, and a resulting injury.

3 Documentation systems

Health care facilities may set their own requirements for documentation and evaluation, but all must comply with legal, accreditation, and professional standards. A nursing department also may select a documentation system, as long as it adheres to those standards.

Depending on your facility's policy, you'll use one or more documentation systems to record your nursing interventions and evaluations and the patient's response. Some facilities use traditional narrative documentation systems. Others choose alternative systems. Each documentation system includes specific policies and procedures for documenting. Understanding and adhering to these requirements will help you to document care systematically and accurately. (See *Comparing documentation systems,* pages 64 to 67.)

Traditional narrative

Narrative documentation is a chronological account of:

- patient's status
- nursing interventions performed
- patient's responses.

Today, few facilities rely on this system alone. Instead, they combine it with other systems, especially the source-oriented record.

FORMAT AND COMPONENTS

In the traditional narrative system, the nurse usually records data as progress notes, with flow sheets supplementing the narrative notes. Knowing when and what to document and how to organize the data are the key elements of effective narrative documenting in the progress notes. (See *Charting in the narrative format.*)

When and what to document

The Joint Commission on Accreditation of Healthcare Organizations (JCAHO) requires all health care facilities to establish policies on the frequency of patient reassessment. Assess your patient at least as often as your facility's policy requires, and then document your findings.

On the other hand, if you find yourself writing repetitious, meaningless notes, you may be documenting too often. If so, double-check your facility's policy. You may be following a time-consuming, unwritten standard initiated by staff members, not by your facility. To guard against this, review the policy at least every 6 months.

In addition to documenting according to facility policy, be sure to write a specific and descriptive narrative in the progress notes whenever you observe any of the following:

- a change in the patient's condition, such as progression, regression, or new

CHART QUICK

Charting in the narrative format

This sample shows how to write progress notes using the narrative system.

Date	Time	Notes
6/26/02	2245	Pt 4 hours postoperative: awakens easily; oriented x 3 but groggy. Incision site in front of Ⓛ ear extending down and around ear and into neck – approximately 6" in length – without dressing. No swelling or bleeding, bluish discoloration below Ⓛ ear noted, sutures intact. Jackson Pratt drain in Ⓛ neck below ear with 20 ml bloody drainage measured. Drain remains secured in place with suture and anchored to Ⓛ anterior chest wall with tape. Pt denied pain but stated she felt nauseated and promptly vomited 100 ml of clear fluid. Pt attempted to get OOB to ambulate to bathroom with assistance but felt dizzy upon standing. Assisted to lie down in bed. Voided 200 ml clear, yellow urine in bedpan. Pt encouraged to deep-breathe and cough q1h and turn frequently in bed. Antiembolism pads applied to both lower extremities. Explanations given re: these preventive measures. Pt verbalized understanding. ——— Bridget Smith, RN
6/26/02	2255	Pt continues to feel nauseated. Compazine 10 mg I.M. given in Ⓡ gluteus maximus. ——— Bridget Smith, RN
6/26/02	2335	Pt states she's no longer nauseated, remains pain free. No further vomiting. Pt demonstrated taking deep breaths and coughing effectively. ——— Bridget Smith, RN

problems. For example, *The patient can ambulate with a walker for 3 minutes before feeling tired.*

- a patient's response to a treatment or medication. For example, *The patient states that abdominal pain is relieved 1 hour after receiving medication. He's smiling and able to turn in bed without difficulty.*
- a lack of improvement in the patient's condition. For example, *No change in size or condition of sacral decubitus ulcer after 6 days of treatment. Dimensions and condition remain as stated in 6/20/02 note.*
- a patient's or family member's response to teaching. For example, *The patient was able to demonstrate walking with crutches using the proper technique.*

Organizing your notes

Before you write anything, organize your thoughts so your paragraphs flow smoothly. If you have trouble deciding

CHART QUICK

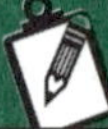

Comparing documentation systems

This table compares elements of the different documentation systems used today. Note that the second column provides information on which systems work best in which settings.

System	Useful settings	Parts of record
Narrative	• Acute care • Long-term care • Home care • Ambulatory care	• Progress notes • Flow sheets to supplement care plan
POMR Problem-oriented medical record	• Acute care • Long-term care • Home care • Rehabilitation • Mental health facilities	• Database • Care plan • Problem list • Progress notes • Discharge summary
PIE Problem-intervention-evaluation	• Acute care	• Assessment flow sheets • Progress notes • Problem list
FOCUS	• Acute care • Long-term care	• Progress notes • Flow sheets • Checklists
CBE Charting by exception	• Acute care • Long-term care	• Care plan • Flow sheets, including patient-teaching records and patient discharge notes • Graphic record • Progress notes
FACT Flow sheet, assessment, concise, timely	• Acute care • Long-term care	• Assessment sheet • Flow sheets • Progress notes

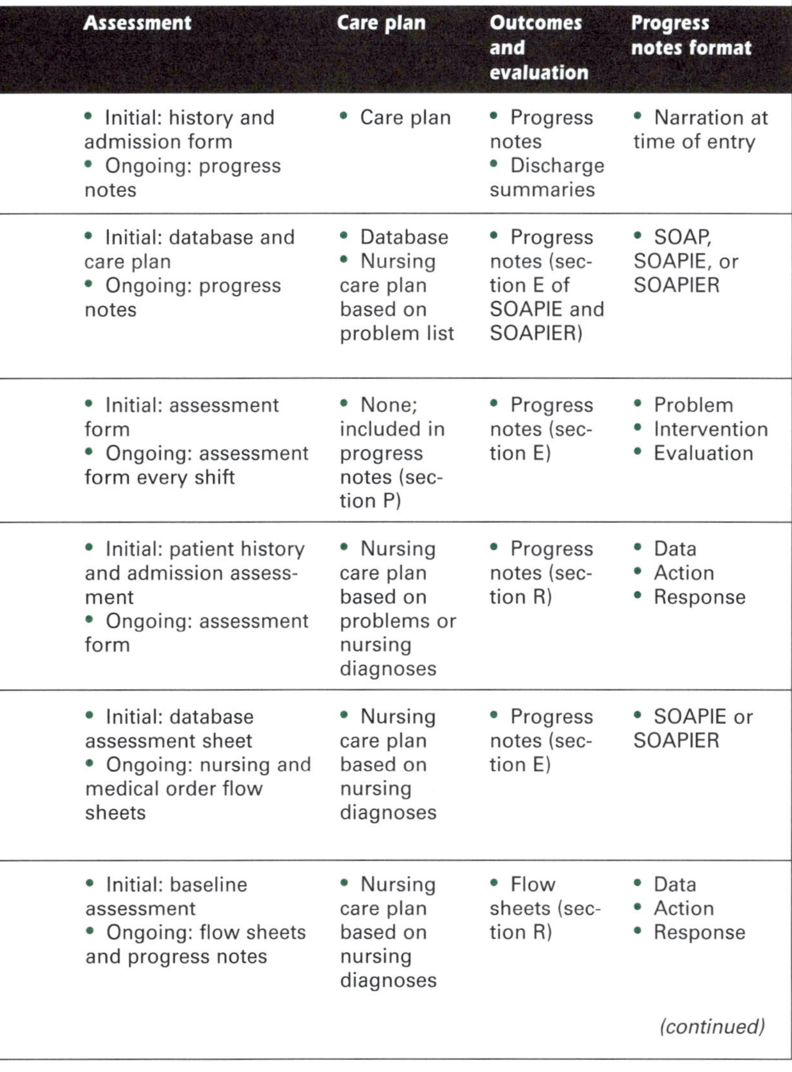

Assessment	Care plan	Outcomes and evaluation	Progress notes format
• Initial: history and admission form • Ongoing: progress notes	• Care plan	• Progress notes • Discharge summaries	• Narration at time of entry
• Initial: database and care plan • Ongoing: progress notes	• Database • Nursing care plan based on problem list	• Progress notes (section E of SOAPIE and SOAPIER)	• SOAP, SOAPIE, or SOAPIER
• Initial: assessment form • Ongoing: assessment form every shift	• None; included in progress notes (section P)	• Progress notes (section E)	• Problem • Intervention • Evaluation
• Initial: patient history and admission assessment • Ongoing: assessment form	• Nursing care plan based on problems or nursing diagnoses	• Progress notes (section R)	• Data • Action • Response
• Initial: database assessment sheet • Ongoing: nursing and medical order flow sheets	• Nursing care plan based on nursing diagnoses	• Progress notes (section E)	• SOAPIE or SOAPIER
• Initial: baseline assessment • Ongoing: flow sheets and progress notes	• Nursing care plan based on nursing diagnoses	• Flow sheets (section R)	• Data • Action • Response

(continued)

Comparing documentation systems *(continued)*

System	Useful settings	Parts of record
Core (with data, action, and evaluation — or DAE)	• Acute care • Long-term care	• Kardex • Flow sheets • Progress notes
Computerized	• Acute care • Long-term care • Home care • Ambulatory care	• Progress notes • Flow sheets • Nursing care plan • Database • Teaching plan

what to write, refer to the patient's care plan to review:

- unresolved problems
- prescribed interventions
- expected outcomes.

Then write down your observations of the patient's progress in these areas. Be sure to include how you first became aware of the problem, what the patient has said about the problem that's significant, your plan for the problem, and the patient's responses to your interventions.

To make your notes as coherent as possible, discuss each of the patient's problems in a separate paragraph. Or, use a head-to-toe approach to organize your information. Be sure to notify the physician of significant changes that you observe. Then document this communication, the physician's responses, and any new orders to be implemented.

A documentation format called AIR may also help you to organize and simplify your narrative documentation. AIR is an acronym for **A**ssessment, **I**ntervention, and **R**esponse. The AIR format synthesizes major nursing events while avoiding repetition of information found elsewhere in the medical record. Combined with nursing flow sheets and the nursing care plan, the AIR format can be used to document clearly and concisely the care you provided.

Here's how AIR is used to document nursing care.

- *Assessment:* Summarize your physical assessment findings. Begin by specifying each issue that you address, such as nursing diagnosis, admission note, and discharge planning. Rather than simply describing the patient's current condition, document trends and record your impression of the problem.
- *Intervention:* Summarize your actions and those of other caregivers in response to the assessment data. The summary may include a condensed nursing care plan or plans for additional patient monitoring.
- *Response:* Summarize the outcome or the patient's response to the nursing interventions. Because a response may

Assessment	Care plan	Outcomes and evaluation	Progress notes format
• Initial: baseline assessment • Ongoing: progress notes	• Care plan	• Progress notes (section E)	• Data • Action • Evaluation
• Initial: baseline assessment • Ongoing: progress notes	• Database • Care plan	• Outcome-based care plan	• Evaluative statements • Expected outcomes • Learning outcomes

not be evident for hours or even days, this documentation may not immediately follow the entries. In fact, it may be recorded by another nurse, which is why titling each of your assessments and interventions is so important.

ADVANTAGES

Narrative documentation offers numerous benefits. This format:

- is the most flexible of all the documentation systems and is suitable in any clinical setting
- strongly conveys your nursing interventions and the patient's responses
- is ideal for presenting information that's collected over a long period
- combines well with other documentation devices, such as flow sheets, which cuts down on documentation time
- uses narration, the most common form of writing, so training new staff members can usually be done quickly
- places its narrative notes in chronological order, so other team members can review the patient's progress daily.

DISADVANTAGES

On the other hand, narrative documentation has the following disadvantages:

- You have to read the entire record to find the patient outcome. Even then, you may have trouble determining the outcome of a problem because the same information may not be consistently documented.
- For the same reason, you may have trouble tracking problems and identifying trends in the patient's progress.
- Narrative documentation offers no inherent guide to what's important to document, so nurses often document everything, resulting in a lengthy, repetitive record.
- Narrative documentation doesn't always reflect the nursing process.
- Narratives may contain vague or inaccurate language, such as "appears to be bleeding" or "small amount."

You may be able to avoid some disadvantages of narrative documentation by organizing the information you record.

Problem-oriented medical record

The problem-oriented medical record (POMR) focuses on specific patient problems and aids communication among team members. It was originally developed by physicians and later adapted by nurses. The POMR is most effective in acute care or long-term care settings.

In this documentation system, you describe each problem in multidisciplinary patient progress notes (not on progress notes with only nursing information).

FORMAT AND COMPONENTS

The POMR is divided into five parts:

- database
- problem list
- initial plan
- progress notes
- discharge summary.

In POMR documentation, you record your interventions and evaluations in the progress notes and discharge summary only. However, to really understand POMR, review all five parts.

Database

Usually completed by a nurse, the database — or initial assessment — is the foundation for the patient's care plan. A collection of subjective and objective information about the patient, the database includes the reason for hospitalization, medical history, allergies, medication regimen, physical and psychosocial findings, self-care abilities, educational needs, and other discharge planning concerns. The database is the basis for a problem list.

Problem list

After analyzing the database, various caregivers list the patient's current problems in chronological order according to the date when each is identified — not in the order of acuteness or priority. This list provides an overview of the patient's health status.

Originally, POMR called for one interdisciplinary problem list. Although this may still be done, nurses and physicians usually keep separate lists with problems stated as either nursing diagnoses or medical diagnoses.

As you list the patient's problems, number them so they correspond to the problems in the rest of the POMR. Have every entry on the patient's initial plan, progress notes, and discharge summary correspond to a number. File the numbered problem list at the front of the patient's chart. Keep the list current by adding new numbers as new problems arise. When writing notes, be sure to identify the problem you're discussing by the appropriate number.

After you have resolved a problem, draw a line through it or show that it's inactive by retiring the problem number and highlighting the problem with a colored felt-tip pen. Don't use that number again for the same patient.

Initial plan

After constructing the problem list, write an initial plan for each problem. This plan includes:

- expected outcomes
- plans for further data collection, if needed
- patient care
- teaching plans.

Involve the patient in goal setting as you construct the initial plan. This fosters the patient's compliance and is essential to the effectiveness of your interventions.

Progress notes

One of the most prominent features of the POMR is the structured way that narrative progress notes are written by all team members using the SOAP, SOAPIE, or SOAPIER format. If you use the SOAP formats, you'll document the following information for each problem:

S: *Subjective data*—information the patient tells you

O: *Objective data*—factual data you gather during assessment

A: *Assessment*—conclusions you reach about the patient's problem based on the subjective and objective information

P: *Plan*—your plan to relieve the patient's problem.

Some facilities use the SOAPIE format, adding:

I: *Intervention*—measures you've taken to achieve a patient outcome

E: *Evaluation*—an analysis of the effectiveness of your interventions.

The SOAPIER format adds a section to document alternative interventions. If your patient's outcomes fall short of expectations, use the evaluation process called for in SOAPIE as a basis for developing revised interventions; then document these changes:

R: *Revision*—document any changes from the original care plan in this section. Interventions, outcomes, or target dates may need to be adjusted to reach a previous goal.

Usually, you must write a complete note in one of these formats every 24 hours whenever a problem is unresolved or the patient's condition changes.

You don't need to write an entry for each SOAP or SOAPIE component every time you document. If you have nothing to record for a component, either omit the letter from the note or leave a blank space after it, depending on your facility's policy. (See *Problem-oriented progress notes,* page 70.)

Discharge summary

The discharge summary—the last part of POMR—covers each problem on the list and notes whether it was resolved. This is the place in your SOAP or SOAPIE note to discuss any unresolved problems and to outline your plan for dealing with the problem after discharge. Also, record communications with other facilities, home health agencies, and the patient.

ADVANTAGES

The POMR charting system has several advantages:

- Information about each problem is organized into specific categories that all caregivers can understand. This eases data retrieval and communication between disciplines.
- Continuity of care is shown by combining the care plan and progress notes into a complete record of care that's planned and care that's delivered. The caregiver addresses each problem or nursing diagnosis in the nurses' notes.
- It encourages nurses to document the nursing process, to document more

CHART QUICK

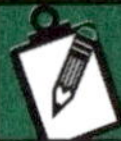

Problem-oriented progress notes

The table below is an example of progress notes as they appear in a problem-oriented medical record. The SOAP framework is used.

Date	Time	Notes
6/7/02	0645	#1 Acute pain
		S: Pt states, "I'm having severe back pain again and
		I'm nauseous."
		O: Pt states pain is #9 on 1 to 10 scale; skin is
		warm, pale, moist. Pt is restless, pacing in room,
		holding R flank area with hand.
		A: Pt in severe pain, needs medication for relief.
		P: Check orders for analgesia; check for any aller-
		gies; take VS; if within normal limits, give analgesia
		as ordered. Recheck pt in 30 minutes for response.
		Monitor pt for adverse reactions to drug. Observe
		pt for pain frequently; offer medication as ordered
		before pain becomes severe. ——— Ann Davis, RN
6/7/02	0657	#1 Acute pain
		S: Pt states, "The pain is less and I'm not nauseous."
		O: Pt states pain is now a #2 on 1 to 10 scale. Skin
		warm, dry, color normal. Pt sitting on bed, watching
		the news.
		A: Pt has improved.
		P: Continue to monitor for pain and other symp-
		toms.
		I: BP 158/84, P 104, RR 24 – morphine sulfate 4 mg
		I.V. given.
		E: Medication was effective. ——— Ann Davis, RN
6/7/02	0730	#2 Anxiety
		S: Pt states, "I'm worried about the surgery and
		being out of work."
		O: Pt wringing hands, eyes downcast.
		A: Pt is anxious regarding upcoming surgery and its
		impact on his job.
		P: Encourage verbalization of feelings and concerns.
		Offer emotional support. Involve family to discuss
		his concerns if agreeable to pt. ——— Ann Davis, RN
6/7/02	0730	#3 Deficient knowledge
		S: Pt states, "I never had surgery before."
		O: Pt is unsure what to expect.
		A: Pt needs preoperative and postoperative educa-
		tion.
		P: Teach pt about events before and after surgery;
		for example, I.V. insertion; teach about the need
		for coughing and deep breathing, moving frequently
		in bed, and early ambulation after surgery. Explain
		why these are important. Evaluate pt's response to
		the teaching, and document. ——— Ann Davis, RN

consistently, and to document only essential data.

- It can be used effectively with standardized care plans and is an integrated medical record.

DISADVANTAGES

The POMR system also has some disadvantages. For example:

- The emphasis on the chronology of problems, rather than their priority, may cause caregivers to disagree about which problems to list.
- Trends may be hard to analyze if information is buried in the daily narrative.
- Assessments and interventions apply to more than one problem, so documenting of these findings is repetitious, especially with the SOAPIE format. This makes documentation time-consuming to perform and to read.
- The format emphasizes problems, so routine care may be left undocumented unless flow sheets are used.
- The format doesn't work well in settings with rapid patient turnover, such as a postanesthesia care unit, a short procedure unit, or an emergency department.
- Problems may arise if caregivers don't keep the problem list current or if they're confused about which problems to list.
- Considerable time and cost is needed to train people to use the SOAP, SOAPIE, and SOAPIER method.

Problem-intervention-evaluation system

The problem-intervention-evaluation (PIE) system organizes information according to patients' problems and was devised to simplify the documentation process.

This system requires you to keep a daily patient assessment flow sheet and write structured progress notes. Integrating the care plan into the nurses' progress notes eliminates the need for a separate care plan. The idea is to provide a concise, efficient record of patient care that has a nursing focus. (See *Using the PIE format,* page 72.)

FORMAT AND COMPONENTS

To use the PIE system, first assess the patient and document your findings on a daily patient assessment flow sheet.

The daily assessment flow sheet lists defined assessment terms under major categories (such as respiration) along with routine care and monitoring measures (such as providing ventilation and monitoring breath sounds). The flow sheet generally includes space to record pertinent treatments.

On the flow sheet, initial only the assessment terms that apply to your patient and mark abnormal findings with an asterisk. Record detailed information in your progress notes.

Next, chart the patient's problems, your interventions, and your evaluations of the patient's responses.

CHART QUICK

Using the PIE format

This sample chart shows how to write progress notes using the problem-intervention-evaluation (PIE) system.

Date	Time	Notes
6/20/02	1300	P#1: Sudden onset of generalized itching and hives possibly related to an allergic reaction.
		IP#1: Note extent of symptoms; take vital signs; assess breath sounds for wheezing. Notify physician immediately. Administer medications as ordered, including I.V. access. Reassure pt.
		EP#1: Symptoms abate; pt maintains adequate respiratory and hemodynamic status; pt verbalized understanding of treatments and need to report further symptoms. — Mary Smith, RN
6/20/02	1300	~~P#2: Ineffective breathing pattern related to possible allergic reaction.~~
		IP#2: Take VS frequently and monitor breath sounds and pulse oximetry. Notify physician for abnormal pulse oximetry or wheezing. Give medications as ordered. Teach pt signs of respiratory distress and the need to report these immediately. — Mary Smith, RN
		EP#2: Pt will have no wheezing or dyspnea; pt verbalized understanding of need to notify nurse of changes in breathing patterns. — Mary Smith, RN

Problem

After performing and documenting an initial assessment, use the collected data to identify pertinent nursing diagnoses. These form the problem piece of PIE. Use the list of nursing diagnoses accepted by your facility, which usually corresponds to the diagnoses approved by the North American Nursing Diagnosis Association (NANDA).

If you can't find a nursing diagnosis on an approved list, write the problem statement yourself using accepted criteria. Make sure you don't use medical diagnoses.

In the progress notes, document all nursing diagnoses or problems, labeling each as *P* and numbering it. For example, the first nursing diagnosis is labeled *P#1*. This way, you can later refer to a specific problem by its label only, without having to redocument the problem statement. Some facilities also use a separate problem-list form to keep a convenient running account of the nursing diagnoses for each patient.

Intervention

To chart the intervention piece of PIE, document the nursing actions you take for each nursing diagnosis. Write them on the progress sheet, labeling each as *I* and assigning the appropriate problem number. For example, to refer to an intervention for the first nursing diagnosis, write *IP#1*.

Evaluation

After charting your interventions, document the patient's responses in your progress notes. These form the evaluation piece of PIE. Use the label *E* followed by the assigned problem number. For example, to identify each evaluation, write *EP#1*.

Make sure that you, or another nurse, evaluate each problem at least once every 8 hours. After every three shifts, review the notes from the previous 24 hours to identify the patient's current problems and responses to interventions.

Document continuing problems daily, along with relevant interventions and evaluations. Cross out resolved problems from the daily documentation.

ADVANTAGES

The PIE format has many attractive features, including:

- ensuring that your documentation includes all of the necessary pieces: nursing diagnoses (problems), related interventions, and evaluations
- providing ongoing documentation of current problems
- encouraging you to meet JCAHO requirements by providing an organized framework for your thoughts and writing
- simplifying documentation by combining the care plan and progress notes and by using the flow sheet for assessment and patient care data
- improving the quality of your progress notes by highlighting interventions and requiring a written evaluation of the patient's response to them.

DISADVANTAGES

The PIE format also has some disadvantages:

- Staff members may need in-depth training before they can use it.
- It requires you to reevaluate each problem once every shift, which is time-consuming and often unnecessary, and leads to repetitive entries.
- It omits documentation of the planning step in the nursing process. This step, which addresses expected outcomes, is essential in evaluating the patient's responses.
- It doesn't incorporate multidisciplinary charting.
- It isn't suitable for long-term care patients.

FOCUS system

Nurses who found the SOAP format awkward developed the FOCUS system of documentation. This system is organized into patient-centered topics, or foci. It encourages you to use assessment data to evaluate these concerns. FOCUS documentation works best in acute care settings and on units where the same care and procedures are repeated frequently.

FORMAT AND COMPONENTS

To implement FOCUS documentation, you'll use a progress sheet with columns for the date, time, focus, and progress notes. You can identify the foci by reviewing your assessment data. (See *Using FOCUS charting,* page 74.)

CHART QUICK

Using FOCUS charting

The table below is an example of progress notes using the FOCUS system.

Date	Time	Focus	Progress notes
6/6/02	1000	Deficient knowledge R/T diagnosis	D: Pt states she doesn't understand what her diagnosis means. A: Illness explained to pt according to her level of understanding. Pt taught symptoms she may expect and why she's having current symptoms. Treatments and procedures explained. Questions answered. Pt encouraged to verbalize need for further instruction or information. R: Pt verbalized better understanding of her illness. — Donna Jones, RN
6/6/02	1000	Risk for deficient fluid volume	D: Pt states her period just began and she's passing a large amount of clots. A: Amount of bleeding assessed. Pt saturated 2 sanitary napkins in the past hour, currently large amount of bright red clots noted. BP 114/70 P 98 RR 20. Pt status reported to physician. Orders received. 20G I.V. catheter started, labs drawn; 1,000 ml NSS hung, macro tubing, at 100 ml/hr. Pt tolerated procedures well. Will continue to monitor vital signs and bleeding. Dr. Smith will be in to see pt. Pt taught how to assess amount of vaginal drainage. R: Pt verbalizes correct amount of drainage and type. Pt understands procedures. — Donna Jones, RN
6/6/02	1000	Anxiety	D: Pt states, "I'm afraid of all this blood." A: Emotional support provided. Encouraged verbalization. Explanations given regarding treatments and procedures. Family in to provide support. R: Pt observed talking and laughing with family. States she feels less anxious. — Donna Jones, RN

Foci

In FOCUS charting, you typically write each focus as a nursing diagnosis, such as *Risk for infection* or *Deficient fluid volume*. However, the focus also may refer to:

- a sign or symptom—such as purulent drainage or chest pain

- a patient behavior — such as an inability to ambulate
- a special need — such as a discharge need
- an acute change in the patient's condition — such as loss of consciousness or increase in blood pressure
- a significant event — such as surgery.

Progress notes

In the progress notes column, identify and divide the information into three categories:

- *data* (D), which include subjective and objective information describing the focus
- *action* (A), which includes immediate and future nursing actions based on your assessment of the patient's condition, as well as changes to the care plan as necessary, based on your evaluation
- *response* (R), which describes the patient's response to nursing or medical care.

Using all three categories guarantees complete documentation based on the nursing process. Be sure to record routine nursing tasks and assessment data on your flow sheets and checklists.

ADVANTAGES

FOCUS documentation has several strong points:

- It's flexible enough to adapt to any clinical setting.
- It centers on the nursing process, and the data-action-response format encourages you to record in a process-oriented way.
- Information on a specific problem is easy to find because the FOCUS statement is separate from the progress note. This promotes communication between health care team members.
- It encourages regular documentation of patient responses to nursing and medical care and ensures adherence to JCAHO requirements.
- You can use this format to document many topics in addition to those on the problem list or care plan.
- It helps you organize your thoughts and document succinctly and precisely.
- It helps you identify areas in the care plan that need revising as you document each entry.

DISADVANTAGES

FOCUS documentation also has weaknesses:

- Staff members — especially those who are used to other systems — may need in-depth training before they can use it.
- You need to use many flow sheets and checklists, which can cause inconsistent documentation and difficulty tracking a patient's problems.
- If you forget to include the patient's response to interventions, FOCUS charting resembles a long narrative such as that seen in progress notes.

Charting by exception

The system called charting by exception (CBE) was designed to eliminate lengthy and repetitive notes, poorly organized information, difficult-to-retrieve data, errors of omission, and other long-standing documentation problems.

To avoid these pitfalls, the CBE format radically departs from traditional systems by requiring documentation of significant or abnormal findings only.

FORMAT AND COMPONENTS

To use CBE effectively, you must adhere to established guidelines for nursing assessments and interventions and follow written standards of practice that identify the nurse's basic responsibilities. Facilities using CBE must have critical pathways or interdisciplinary care plans that address every possible patient problem.

Guidelines for each body system are printed on CBE forms. For example, care standards for patient hygiene might specify a complete linen change every 3 days or sooner, if necessary. Having the standards clearly and concisely written eliminates the need to document routine nursing care or any other care outlined in the standards — all you document are deviations from the standards.

Guidelines for interventions used in the CBE system come from these sources:

- *nursing diagnosis–based standardized care plans.* These identify patient problems, desired outcomes, and interventions.
- *patient care guidelines.* These are standardized interventions created for specific patients, such as those with a nursing diagnosis of acute or chronic pain. These guidelines outline the nursing interventions, treatments, and time frame for repeated assessments.
- *physician's orders.* These are prescribed medical interventions.
- *incidental orders.* These are usually one-time, miscellaneous nursing or medical orders or interdependent interventions related to a protocol or a piece of equipment.
- *standards of nursing practice.* These define the acceptable level of routine nursing care for all patients. They may describe the essential aspects of nursing practice for a specific unit or for all clinical areas.

The CBE format includes a standardized care plans based on the nursing diagnosis and several types of flow sheets. These flow sheets include:

- nursing and medical order flow sheet
- graphic form
- patient-teaching record
- patient discharge note.

Sometimes you may need to supplement your CBE documentation by using nurses' progress notes.

Standardized care plans

Using the CBE format for documentation involves filling out a preprinted care plans for each nursing diagnosis. These preprinted plans have blank spaces so you can individualize them as needed. For example, include expected outcomes and major revisions in your care plans. Place the completed forms in the nurses' progress notes section of the clinical record.

Nursing and medical order flow sheets

Use nursing and medical order flow sheets to document your assessments and interventions. Each flow sheet covers a 24-hour period of care for one patient.

The top part of the flow sheet contains the physician's orders for assessments and interventions. Each nursing order includes a corresponding nursing diagnosis, labeled *ND #1, ND #2,* and so on; physician's orders are labeled

CHART QUICK

Using a nursing and medical order flow sheet

Here are the typical features of a nursing and medical order flow sheet.

NURSING AND MEDICAL ORDER FLOW SHEET

Date 5/22/02

ND #/DO	Assessment and interventions		
ND 1	Wound assessment	0700*	1500*
ND 2	Range of motion assessment		
DO	Ancef 2 g I.V. stat x 1/1 dose	0645√	
Initials		CF	CF

Key DO = doctor's orders
ND = nursing diagnosis
√ = normal findings
➔ = no change in condition
* = abnormal or significant finding (see Comments section)

ND #/DO	Time	Comments	Initials
ND 1	0800	Ⓡ leg wound with yellow drainage, inflammation around border. Physician notified. No complaint of pain.	CF
ND 1	0830	Pt able to move both lower extremities 1" off bed.	CF
ND 1	1100	No drainage on Ⓡ leg dressing	CF
ND 2	1100	Pt rates pain decreased to a 3/10	CF

Initials CF **Signature** Cary Filiano, RN

DO. (See *Using a nursing and medical order flow sheet*.)

In addition to the abbreviations, *ND* for "nursing diagnosis" and *DO* for "doctor's orders," use these symbols when you record care on flow sheets:

- a check mark (✔) to indicate a completed medical order or nursing assessment with no abnormal findings
- an asterisk (✻) to indicate an abnormal finding on an assessment or an abnormal response to an intervention
- an arrow (➔) to indicate that the patient's status hasn't changed since the previous entry.

ASSESSMENT

After completing an assessment, compare your findings with the printed guidelines on the back of the form. If a finding is within normal parameters, place a check mark in the appropriate box. If a finding isn't within the normal range, put an asterisk in the box. Then explain your findings in the comments section on the form.

An assessment finding that isn't defined in the guidelines may be normal for a particular patient. For example, unclear speech may be normal in a patient with a long-standing tracheostomy. Reference this type of note by nursing diagnosis number or doctor's order and time. If the patient's condition hasn't changed from the last assessment, draw a horizontal arrow from the previous category box to the current one.

INTERVENTIONS

Document interventions similarly. Use a check mark to indicate a completed intervention and an expected patient response. Indicate significant findings or abnormal patient responses with an asterisk, and write an explanation in the comments section. When the patient's response is unchanged, use an arrow.

After you document an entire column in the assessments and interventions section, initial it at the bottom. Also, initial all of your entries in the comments section, and sign the form at the bottom of the page.

COMBINATION FLOW SHEETS

Some facilities use a special nursing care flow sheet that combines all of the necessary forms, such as the graphic record, the daily activities checklist, and the patient care assessment section. (See *Using a combined nursing care flow sheet.*)

Graphic form

The graphic form section of a flow sheet is used to document trends in the patient's vital signs, weight, intake and output, and stool, urination, appetite, and activity levels.

As with the nursing and medical order flow sheet, use check marks to indicate expected findings and use asterisks to indicate abnormal ones. Record information about abnormalities in the nurses' progress notes or on the nursing and medical order flow sheet.

In the box labeled "routine standards," check off the nursing care interventions you performed, such as providing hygiene. Don't rewrite these standards as orders on the nursing and medical order flow sheet. Refer to the guidelines on the back of the graphic form for complete instructions.

Patient-teaching record

Use the patient-teaching form (or section) to identify the information, psychomotor skills, and social or behavioral measures that your patient or his caregiver must learn by a predetermined date.

This record includes teaching resources, dates of patient achievements, and other pertinent observations. If the patient has multiple learning needs, you can use more than one form.

Patient discharge note

Like other discharge forms, the patient discharge note is a flow sheet for documenting ongoing discharge planning. To chart discharge planning, follow the instructions printed on the back of the form. A typical discharge note includes patient instructions, appointments for follow-up care, medication and diet instructions, signs and symptoms to report, level of activity, and wound care.

Progress notes

Use the progress notes to document revisions in the care plans and interventions that don't lend themselves to the nursing and medical order flow sheet. Because the CBE format allows you to document most assessments and interventions on the nursing and medical order flow sheet, your progress notes usually contain little assessment and intervention data.

(Text continues on page 82.)

CHART QUICK

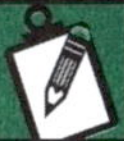

Using a combined nursing care flow sheet

This sample shows a portion of a nursing care flow sheet that combines a graphic record, a daily nursing care activities checklist, and a patient care assessment form.

24-HOUR NURSING CARE FLOW SHEET

Name Maureen Galen

Date	6/29/02											
Hour	0700	0800	0900	1000	1100	1200	1300	1400	1500	1600	1700	1800
Temperature												
°C °F												
40.4 105												
40.0 104												
39.4 103												
38.9 102												
37.8 100												
37.2 99												
36.7 98												
36.1 97												
35.6 96												
Pulse	84	80	82	78	76	78	78	82	84	82	80	78
Respiration	16	20	20	22	24	24	18	20	22	20	18	24
BP Lying												
Sitting	136/82	130/80	126/74	132/82	132/80	140/82	136/74	130/70	138/78	140/80	132/78	136/76
Standing												

Intake		
Oral	240 360	120
Tube		
I.V.		
Blood		
8-hour total	600	
Output	400 450	
Other		
8-hour total	850	
Teaching	dressing changes, s/s of infection	
Signature	Mary Murphy, RN	Ann Burns, RN

(continued)

Using a combined nursing care flow sheet (continued)

	Hour	0700	0800	0900	1000	1100	1200	1300	1400	1500	1600	1700
ACTIVITY	Bedrest	MM →								AB →		
	OOB											
	Ambulate (assist)											
	Ambulatory											
	Sleeping											
	Bathroom privileges											
	HOB elevated	MM →								AB →		
	Cough, deep breathe, turn		MM								AB	
	ROM Active		MM								AB	
	ROM Passive											
HYGIENE	Bath		MM									
	Shave		MM									
	Oral		MM									
	Skin care											
	Peri care											
NUTRITION	Diet		House									
	% eating			75%			60%					75%
	Feeding											
	Supplemental											
	S-Self A-Assist F-Feed		A				A					A
BLADDER	Catheter		indwelling urinary #18 Fr.									
	Incontinent											
	Voiding		clear, yellow urine									
	Intermittent catheter											
BOWEL	Stools (occult blood + or –)											
	Incontinent											
	Normal		large formed brown stool									
	Enema											
SPECIAL TREATMENTS	Special mattress		Low pressure airflow mattress applied 0900									
	Special bed											
	Heel and elbow pads											
	Antiembolism stockings											
	Traction: + = on, – = off											
	Isolation type											

Using a combined nursing care flow sheet *(continued)*

ASSESSMENT FINDINGS

Key
√ = normal findings
* = significant findings

	Day	Evening	Night	
Neurologic	* MM	√ AB		0800 Limited ROM L shoulder, Pt states "I have arthritis and my shoulder is always stiff"
Cardiovascular (CV)	√ MM	√ AB		
Respiratory	√ MM	* AB		1800 shallow breathing with poor respiratory effort at 1700
GI	√ MM	√ AB		
Genitourinary (GU)	√ MM	√ AB		
Surgical dressing and incision	* MM	√ AB		0930 incision reddened; dime-sized area of serous sanguineous drainage on old dressing
Skin integrity	√ MM	√ AB		
Psychosocial	√ MM	√ AB		
Educational	* MM	√ AB		0945 Taught pt incisional care and dressing change, and s/s of infection
Peripheral vascular	√ MM	√ AB		

NORMAL ASSESSMENT FINDINGS

Neurologic assessment
- Alert and oriented to person, place, and time
- Speech clear and understandable
- Memory intact
- Behavior appropriate to situation and accommodation
- Active range of motion (ROM) of all extremities, symmetrically equal strength
- No paresthesia

Cardiovascular assessment
- Regular apical pulse
- Palpable bilateral peripheral pulses
- No peripheral edema
- No calf tenderness

Pulmonary assessment
- Resting respirations 10 to 20 per minute, quiet and regular
- Clear sputum
- Pink nailbeds and mucous membranes

GI assessment
- Abdomen soft and nondistended
- Tolerates prescribed diet without nausea or vomiting
- Bowel movements within own normal pattern and consistency (as described in Patient Profile)

GU assessment
- No indwelling catheter in use
- Urinates without pain
- Undistended bladder after urination
- Urine is clear, yellow to amber color

Surgical dressing and incision assessment
- Dressing dry and intact
- No evidence of redness, increased temperature, or tenderness in surrounding tissue
- Sutures, staples, or Steri-Strips intact
- Wound edges well-approximated
- No drainage present

(continued)

Using a combined nursing care flow sheet *(continued)*

NORMAL ASSESSMENT FINDINGS *(continued)*

Skin integrity assessment
- Skin color normal
- Skin warm, dry, and intact
- Moist mucous membranes

Psychosocial assessment
- Interacts and communicates in an appropriate manner with others (family, significant others, health care personnel)

Educational assessment
- Patient or significant others communicate understanding of the patient's health status, care plan, and expected response
- Patient or significant others demonstrate ability to perform health-related procedures and behaviors as taught
- Items taught and expected performance must be specifically described in Significant Findings Section

Peripheral vascular assessment
- Affected extremity is pink, warm, and movable within average ROM
- Capillary refill time less than 3 seconds
- Peripheral pulses palpable
- No edema, sensation intact without numbness or paresthesia
- No pain on passive stretch

ADVANTAGES

The CBE format has several benefits:

- It eliminates documentation of routine care through the use of nursing care standards. This stops redundancies and clearly identifies abnormal data.
- CBE is easily adapted to documentation on clinical pathways.
- Information that has already been recorded isn't repeated. For instance, you don't have to write a long entry each time you assess a patient whose condition has stayed the same.
- The use of well-defined guidelines and standards of care promotes uniform nursing practice.
- The flow sheets let you track trends easily.
- Guidelines are printed on the forms for ready reference. Abnormal findings are highlighted to help you quickly pinpoint significant changes and trends in a patient's condition.
- Patient data are immediately written on the permanent record. Because you don't need to keep temporary notes and then transcribe them in the patient's chart later, all caregivers always have access to the most current data, which decreases documentation time.
- Assessments are standardized so all caregivers evaluate and document findings consistently.
- All flow sheets are kept at the patient's bedside, where they serve as a ready reference. This encourages immediate documentation.

DISADVANTAGES

Drawbacks of the CBE system include the following:

- The development of clear guidelines and standards of care is time-consuming. For legal reasons, these guidelines and standards must be written and understood by all nurses before the system can be implemented.
- This system takes a long time for people to learn, accept, and use correctly and consistently.

- Duplicate documentation occurs with CBE; nursing diagnoses on a problem list are also written on the care plan.
- Narrative notes and evaluations of patients' responses may be brief and sketchy in facilities that use multiple forms instead of one combination form.
- This system was developed for RNs. Before LPNs can use it, it must be evaluated and modified to meet their scope of practice.

FACT system

The computer-ready FACT documentation system incorporates many CBE principles. It was developed to help caregivers avoid the documentation of irrelevant data, repetitive notes, and inconsistencies among departments and to reduce the time spent charting.

FORMAT AND COMPONENTS

The FACT system has four key elements:

- Flow sheets individualized to specific services
- Assessment features standardized with baseline parameters
- Concise, integrated progress notes and flow sheets documenting the patient's condition and responses
- Timely entries recorded when care is given.

In this system, you document only exceptions to the norm or significant information about the patient.

The FACT format uses an assessment and action flow sheet, a frequent assessment flow sheet, and progress notes. The content of flow sheets and notes may be individualized to some extent. The flow sheets cover a 24- to 72-hour time span, and you need to date, time, and sign all entries. (See *Documenting with the FACT system,* pages 84 and 85.)

Assessment and action flow sheet

Use the assessment and action flow sheet to document ongoing assessments and interventions. Normal assessment parameters for each body system are printed on the form, along with the planned interventions. You may individualize the flow sheet according to the patient's needs.

Frequent assessment flow sheet

The frequent assessment flow sheet is where you chart vital signs and frequent assessments. On a surgical unit, for example, this form would include a postoperative assessment section.

Progress notes

The FACT system requires an integrated progress record. Use narrative notes to document the patient's progress and any significant incidents. As in FOCUS documentation, write narrative notes using the data-action-response method. Update progress notes related to patient outcomes every 48 hours.

ADVANTAGES

The FACT charting system has many good points. For example, this system:

- eliminates repetition and encourages consistent language and structure
- eliminates detailed documentation of normal findings and incorporates each step of the nursing process
- is outcome oriented and communicates the patient's progress to all health care team members

(Text continues on page 86.)

CHART QUICK

Documenting with the FACT system

This sample shows portions of an assessment flow sheet and a postoperative flow sheet using the FACT format.

ASSESSMENT RECORD

Date / Time	6/18/02 0100	6/18/02 0500	6/18/02 0900
Neurologic Alert and oriented to time, place, and person. PERLA. Symmetry of strength in extremities. No difficulty with coordination. Behavior appropriate to situation. Sensation intact without numbness or paresthesia.	✓	✓	✓
Orient patient.			
Refer to neurologic flow sheet.			
Pain No report of pain. If present, include patient statements about intensity (0 to 5 scale), location, description, duration, radiation, precipitating and alleviating factors.	5-Neck pain	✓	7-Neck pain "It hurts."
Location	Cervical spine area		Cervical spine area
Relief measures	Pt repositioned		Percocet † p.o.
Pain relief: Yes/No	Y		Y
Cardiac Apical pulse 60 to 100. S_1 and S_2 present. Regular rhythm. Peripheral (radial, pedal) pulses present. No edema or calf tenderness. Extremities pink, warm, movable within patient's ROM.	✓	✓	✓
I.V. solution and rate	D_5½ NSS @ KVO	D_5½ NSS @ KVO	D_5½ NSS @ KVO
Pulmonary Respiratory rate 12 to 20 at rest, quiet, regular and nonlabored. Lungs clear and aerated equally in all lobes. No SOB at rest. No abnormal lung sounds. Mucous membranes pink.	✓	✓	✓
O_2 therapy			
Taught coughing, deep breathing, incentive spirometer	✓	✓	✓
Musculoskeletal Extremities pink, warm, and without edema; sensation and motion present. Normal joint ROM, no swelling or tenderness. Steady gait without aids. Pedal, radial pulses present. Rapid capillary refill.	✓	✓	✓
Activity (describe)	bed rest	OOB in chair	bed rest
Nurse's signature and title	Jane Doe, RN	Jane Doe, RN	Jane Doe, RN

Key: ✓ Meets assessment criteria

Documenting with the FACT system *(continued)*

POSTOPERATIVE RECORD

Hour	1100	1115	1130	1145		
Blood pressure V:Systolic	140	135	130	140		
Blood pressure Λ:Diastolic	80	80	80	80		
Temperature	36.8	37	37	36.7		
Pulse Apical	80	72	72	70		
Pulse Radial	80	76	78	72		
Respiration	18	20	18	17		
Sedation	2	2	2	2		
Pain	2	3	2	2		
Dressing and site	✓	✓	✓	✓		
Skin	✓	✓	✓	✓		
Peripheral pulse	✓	✓	✓	✓		
CNS	✓	✓	✓	✓		
Deep breathing	✓	✓	✓	✓		
Other						
Initials	EJ	EJ	EJ	EJ		

(Blood pressure scale: 220, 210, 200, 190, 180, 170, 160, 150, 140, 130, 120, 110, 100, 90, 80, 70, 60, 50, 40)

Date 6/18/02

Procedure Cervical myelogram

Tubes and drains none

KEY AND GUIDELINES

Sedation scale

1 Alert. Able to converse or track with eyes.
2 Sleepy. Easy to arouse.
3 Lethargic. Difficult to arouse.
4 Responds only to maximal stimulation.
5 Unable to respond.
AS Asleep at time.

Pain scale

Patient rates pain on scale of
0 (no pain) to **5** (unbearable).
AS Asleep at time.
NA Not able to assess. Patient unable to describe.

Dressing and site

✓ Normal — flat, intact, dry minimal drainage
* Abnormal — drainage, ecchymosis

Skin

✓ Normal — warm, dry, pink
* Abnormal

Peripheral pulse

✓ Present
* Abnormal — absent or weak

CNS

✓ Normal
* Abnormal

Deep breathing

✓ Done
* Document abnormal findings on assessment flow sheet

Initials	Signature and title
EJ	Ellen Johnson, RN

- permits immediate recording of current data and is readily accessible at the patient's bedside
- eliminates the need for many different forms and reduces the time spent writing narrative notes
- is cost effective.

DISADVANTAGES

FACT documentation does have some problems:

- Development of standards and implementation of a facility-wide system require a major time commitment.
- Narrative notes may be sketchy, and the nurse's perspective on the patient may be overlooked.
- The nursing process framework may be difficult to identify.

Core system

The Core system focuses on the nursing process, which is the core of documentation. It's most useful in acute care and long-term care facilities.

FORMAT AND COMPONENTS

The Core system requires you to assess and record a patient's functional and cognitive status within 8 hours of admission. It consists of:

- database
- care plan
- flow sheets
- progress notes
- discharge summary.

Database

The database (initial assessment form) focuses on the patient's body systems and activities of daily living. It includes a summary of his problems and appropriate nursing diagnoses. The nurse enters the completed database onto the patient's medical record card or Kardex.

Care plan

The completed care plan (like the database) goes on the patient's medical record card or Kardex.

Flow sheets

Use flow sheets to document the patient's activities and his response to nursing interventions, diagnostic procedures, and patient teaching.

Progress notes

On the progress notes sheet, record the DAE — data (D), action (A), and evaluation (E) or response — for each problem.

Discharge summary

The discharge summary includes information about the nursing diagnoses, patient teaching, and recommended follow-up care.

ADVANTAGES

The Core with DAE documentation system offers several advantages:

- It incorporates the entire nursing process.
- The DAE component helps to ensure complete documentation based on the nursing process.
- It encourages concise documenting with minimal repetition.
- It allows the daily recording of psychosocial information.

DISADVANTAGES

Core documentation has several disadvantages:

- Staff members who are used to other documenting systems may need in-depth training.
- Development of forms may be costly and time-consuming.
- The DAE format doesn't always present information chronologically, making it difficult to quickly perceive the patient's progress.
- The progress notes may not always relate to the care plan, so you need to monitor carefully to make sure the record shows high-quality care.

Computerized documentation

Computerization can significantly reduce the time you spend on documentation and increase your accuracy. Computers can also be used to help you with other types of paperwork, such as:

- nurse management reports
- patient classification data
- staffing projections.

In addition, they can help you identify patient education needs and supply data for nursing research and education. Some bedside terminals can even measure vital signs.

In addition to having a mainframe computer, most health care facilities place personal computers or terminals at workstations throughout the facility so departmental staff will have quick access to vital information. Some facilities put terminals at patients' bedsides, making data even more easily accessible.

Before entering a patient's clinical record into a computer, you must first enter a special code, which is usually your computer ID number. Some codes may specify the type of information to which a particular team member has access. For example, a dietitian may be assigned a code that allows her to see dietary orders and nutrition histories but not physical therapy information. These codes can help maintain a patient's privacy, unless they're misused.

Here's how to use a computerized system for documentation: First, enter the special code, the patient's name, or his account number to bring the patient's electronic chart to the screen. Then choose the function you want to perform.

For example, you can enter new data on the nursing care plan or progress notes or scan the record to compare data on vital signs or intake and output. Usually, you can obtain information more quickly with computers than with traditional documentation systems.

COMPUTER SYSTEMS AND FUNCTIONS

Depending on which type of computer and software your facility has, you may access information by using your voice, a keyboard, a light pen, a touch-sensitive screen, or a mouse.

Specialized nursing information systems can increase your efficiency in all phases of documentation. Most provide a menu of words or phrases you can choose from to individualize your documentation on standardized forms. With some computerized systems, you can use a series of phrases to quickly create a complete narrative note. Then you can elaborate on a problem or clarify flow sheet documentation in the comment section of a computerized form by entering standardized phrases or typing in comments. Important developments in computer systems include specialized nursing information systems (NISs), the nursing minimum data set (NMDS), and voice-activated systems. (See *Computers and the nursing process*.)

Nursing information systems

Currently available NIS software programs allow you to record nursing actions in the electronic record, making documentation easier. These systems reflect most or all of the components of the nursing process so they can meet the standards of the American Nurses Association and JCAHO. Furthermore, each NIS provides different features and can be customized to conform to a facility's documentation forms and formats. NISs can link nursing resources to educational applications.

At present, most NISs manage information passively — that is, they collect, transmit, organize, format, print, and display information that you can use to make a decision, but they don't suggest decisions for you.

NEW DEVELOPMENTS

The most current NISs interact with you, prompting you with questions and suggestions about the information you enter. Ultimately, this computerized, sequential decision-making format should lead to more effective nursing care and documentation.

An interactive system requires you to enter only a brief narrative. The questions and suggestions the computer program provides make your documentation thorough and quick. The program also allows you to add or change information so that your documentation fits your patient.

Nursing minimum data set

The NMDS program attempts to standardize nursing information. It contains three categories of data:

- nursing care, such as nursing diagnoses and interventions
- patient demographics, such as the patient's name, birth date, gender, race and ethnicity, and residence
- service elements such as length of hospitalization.

NURSING BENEFITS

The NMDS documentation system allows you to collect nursing diagnoses and intervention data and to identify the nursing needs of various patient populations. It lets you track patient outcomes and describe nursing care in different settings, including the patient's home. It also helps establish accurate estimates for nursing service costs and provides data about nursing care that may influence health care policy and decision making.

In addition, you can compare nursing trends locally, regionally, and nationally and compare nursing data from various clinical settings, patient populations, and geographic areas.

The NMDS also helps you provide better patient care. For instance, examining the outcomes of patient populations will help you set realistic outcomes for an individual patient. This system also can help you develop accurate nursing diagnoses and plan interventions.

The standardized format encourages more consistent nursing documentation. All data are coded, making documentation and information retrieval faster and easier. Currently, NANDA assigns numerical codes to all nursing

Computers and the nursing process

A computer information system can either stand alone or be a subsystem of a larger hospital system. Nursing information systems (NISs) can increase efficiency and accuracy in all phases of the nursing process — assessment, nursing diagnosis, planning, implementation, and evaluation — and can help nurses meet the standards established by the American Nurses Association and the Joint Commission on Accreditation of Healthcare Organizations. In addition, an NIS can help you spend more time meeting the patient's needs. Consider the following uses of computers in the nursing process.

Assessment

Use the computer terminal to record admission information. As you collect data, enter further information as prompted by the computer's software program. Enter data about the patient's health status, history, chief complaint, and other assessment factors.

Some software programs prompt you to ask specific questions and then offer pathways to gather further information. In some systems, if you enter an assessment value that's outside the usual acceptable range, the computer will flag the entry to call your attention to it.

Nursing diagnosis

Most current programs list standard diagnoses with associated signs and symptoms as references. But you must still use clinical judgment to determine a nursing diagnosis for each patient. With this information, you can rapidly obtain diagnostic information.

For example, the computer can generate a list of possible diagnoses for a patient with selected signs and symptoms, or it may enable you to retrieve and review the patient's records according to the nursing diagnosis.

Planning

To help nurses begin writing a care plan, newer computer programs display recommended expected outcomes and interventions for the selected diagnoses. Computers can also track outcomes for large patient populations.

You can use computers to compare large amounts of patient data, help identify outcomes the patient is likely to achieve based on individual problems and needs, and estimate the time frame for reaching outcome goals.

Implementation

Use the computer to record actual interventions and patient-processing information, such as transfer and discharge instructions, and to communicate this information to other departments. Computer-generated progress notes automatically sort and print out patient data — such as medication administration, treatments, and vital signs — making documentation more efficient and accurate.

Evaluation

During evaluation, use the computer to record and store observations, patient responses to nursing interventions, and your own evaluation statements. You may also use information from other members of the health care team to determine future actions and discharge planning. If a desired patient outcome hasn't been achieved, record new interventions taken to ensure desired outcomes. Then reevaluate the second set of interventions.

diagnoses so they can be used with the NMDS.

Voice-activated systems

Some facilities have voice-activated nursing documentation systems. These are most useful in departments that have a high volume of structured reports, such as the operating room.

This system uses a specialized knowledge base of nursing words, phrases, and report forms combined with automated speech recognition technology. You can record nurses' notes by voice, promptly and completely. The system requires little or no keyboard use — you simply speak into a telephone handset, and the text appears on the computer screen.

The software program includes information on the nursing process, nursing theory, nursing standards of practice, and report forms in a logical format. Trigger phrases cue the system to display passages of report text. You can use the text displayed to design an individualized care plan or to fill in standard hospital forms.

Although voice-activated systems work most efficiently with trigger phrases, word-for-word dictation and editing are possible. The system increases the nurse's recording speed and decreases paperwork.

ADVANTAGES

Most nurses have good things to say about computerized documentation:

- It makes storing and retrieving information fast and easy.
- You can store data on patient populations that can help improve the quality of nursing care.
- You can efficiently and constantly update information and help link diverse sources of patient information.
- It uses standard terminology, which improves communication among health care disciplines and promotes more accurate comparisons.
- The documentation is always legible.
- You can send request slips and patient information from one terminal to another quickly and efficiently, which helps ensure confidentiality.
- It facilitates individualized patient assessments and supports the use of the nursing process.

DISADVANTAGES

However, computerized documentation also has shortcomings:

- If used incorrectly, the computer may scramble patient information.
- Computerized documentation can threaten patient confidentiality if security measures are neglected.
- The use of standardized phrases and a limited vocabulary can make information inaccurate or incomplete.
- Some people have trouble adjusting to computers, thus increasing the margin for error.
- During times of peak use, processing can be slow, and during computer servicing time or computer failure, patient information may be temporarily unavailable.
- Computer documentation can take extra time if too many nurses try to chart on too few terminals.
- Implementing a computerized documentation system is expensive.
- Software that puts patient data into categories may cause important information to be omitted.

Choosing a documentation system

Health care facilities are always striving for greater efficiency and quality of care. A top-notch charting system can help a facility reach these goals.

Remember, documentation is often examined to make sure a facility meets the profession's minimum acceptable level of care. If efficiency and quality levels are low, your charting system may need to be modified or replaced.

Continuous quality improvement programs are mandated by the state and JCAHO. Committees that set up these programs choose well-defined, objective, and easily measurable indicators that help them assess the structure, process, and outcome of patient care. They also use these indicators to monitor and evaluate the contents of a patient's medical record.

Shorter hospital stays and the requirement to verify the need for supplies and equipment have placed greater emphasis on nursing documentation as a yardstick for measuring the quality of patient care and determining whether it was required and provided.

To verify that treatment was required and provided or that medical tests and supplies were used, the insurers (also called third-party payers) review nursing documentation carefully. As a result, nurses now need to document more information than ever before, including every I.V. needle used to start an infusion, each use of an I.V. pump to deliver a specific volume of medication, and every test that the patient undergoes.

When changes are called for, you may be asked to serve on a committee that decides whether your documentation system needs a simple revision or a total overhaul. Before committing to a totally new system, your committee will discuss the possibility of revising the current system. This, of course, is easier than switching to a new system and changing the way information is collected, entered, and retrieved. To help you and your committee decide whether to revise your current system or change to a new system, consider the following questions:

- What are the specific positive features of our current documentation system?
- What are the specific problems or limitations of our current system? How can they be resolved?
- How much time will we need to develop a new system, educate the staff, and implement the changes?
- Will a new system be cost effective?
- How will changing the documentation system affect other members of the health care team, including the business office staff and medical staff?
- How will we handle resistance to the proposed changes?

When choosing a new documentation system, consider the type of care that's provided at your facility. For example, some systems work better in acute care than in long-term care settings.

Cost is another important factor to consider. Although computer systems are used in almost every care setting, the cost of a new system can be astronomical—all the more reason to weigh the options very carefully.

If a new documentation system is selected, staff will require plenty of training. The system may be initiated on one unit at a time to make the transition easier.

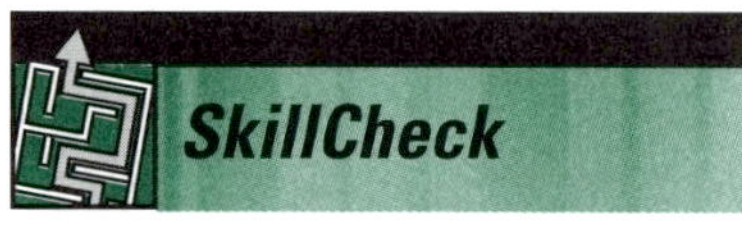

1. Which documentation format calls for you to record only abnormal findings?

a. FOCUS
b. CBE
c. PIE
d. Narrative

Answer: b. CBE departs from other documentation systems by requiring documentation of only significant or abnormal findings.

2. Which documentation format uses the SOAPIE method?

a. POMR
b. FOCUS
c. PIE
d. FACT

Answer: a. A prominent feature of the POMR is the structured way that the narrative notes are written using the SOAP, SOAPIE, or SOAPIER format.

3. In the SOAP documentation method, you would include a patient's complaint about a leaking dressing under which of the following?

a. S
b. O
c. A
d. P

Answer: a. The patient's complaint would fall under subjective data—information the patient tells you—and should be documented under S.

4. If you're documenting data, action, and evaluation, you're using:

a. FOCUS documentation
b. FACT documentation
c. PIE documentation
d. Core documentation

Answer: d. The DAE component of Core documentation helps to ensure complete documentation based on the nursing process.

5. In the PIE documentation format, where would you include the statement *Administered Demerol and assisted with repositioning from back to left side?*

a. P
b. I
c. E
d. You wouldn't include this statement in PIE documentation

Answer: b. You would document your nursing actions under the intervention piece of PIE.

4 Documenting in acute care

Like many nurses working in acute care settings, you may feel discouraged — even overwhelmed — by the amount of information you have to document each day. You may also be baffled by new methods of documentation, such as computer documenting, flow sheets, and critical pathways. Ironically, formats that are meant to save time for nurses may actually end up costing time. Nurses accustomed to writing long, handwritten notes may be uncomfortable taking advantage of shortcuts offered by newer methods, especially given today's litigious environment, in which documentation is strongly linked to liability. The result: Many nurses end up double-documenting — for example, recording the information with a check mark on a flow sheet and then documenting it again in longhand in progress notes.

To cope with the documentation chaos that characterizes contemporary nursing, your best weapon is familiarity with the variety of formats available, their advantages and disadvantages, and how you can use them to enhance your nursing practice.

The following forms — commonly used to create medical records in acute care settings — are explained in this chapter:

- admission database or admission assessment forms
- nursing care plans
- critical pathways
- patient care Kardexes
- graphic forms
- progress notes
- flow sheets
- discharge summary and patient discharge instruction forms.

Other forms include patient-teaching documents, dictated documentation, and patient self-documentation. Adapted or newly developed forms also may be used.

A medical record with well-organized, completed forms serves three purposes:

- It helps you to communicate patient information to other members of the health care team.
- It protects you and your employer legally by providing evidence of the nature and quality of care the patient received.
- It's used by your facility to obtain accreditation and reimbursement for care.

In the long run, taking the time to carefully commit patient information to a standard, easy-to-use format frees you to spend more time on direct patient care.

Admission database form

The admission database form—also known as an admission assessment—is used to document your initial patient assessment. The scope of information documented at this stage is usually broad because you're establishing a comprehensive base of clinical information.

The Joint Commission on Accreditation of Healthcare Organizations (JCAHO) requires that the admission assessment—including a health history and physical examination—be completed within 24 hours of admission; some facilities require a shorter time frame. To complete the admission database form, you must collect relevant information from various sources and analyze it. The finished form portrays a complete picture of the patient at admission.

The admission database form may be organized in different ways. Some facilities use a form organized by body system. Others use a format that groups information to reflect such principles of nursing practice as patient response patterns.

More facilities are using integrated admission database forms. On an integrated admission database form, nursing and medical assessments complement each other, reducing the need for repeated documentation. (See *Integrated admission database form.*)

Regardless of how the form is organized, findings are documented in two basic styles:

- standardized, open-ended style, which comes with preprinted headings and questions
- standardized, closed-ended style, which has preprinted headings, checklists, and questions with specific responses (you simply check off the appropriate response). Most facilities use a combination of styles in one form.

As you complete the admission database form, keep in mind that the information you document is used by JCAHO, quality improvement groups, and other parties to continue accreditation, justify requests for reimbursement, and maintain or improve patient care standards.

A carefully completed admission database form is extremely valuable. It contains physiologic, psychosocial, and cultural information that's useful throughout the patient's stay in your facility. It provides:

- baseline data that's used later for comparison with the patient's progress
- important information about the patient's current health status as well as clues about actual and potential health problems (for example, your admission assessment may turn up facts about prescription and over-the-counter drugs the patient takes; possible drug allergies also may be revealed)
- insight into the patient's ability to comply with therapy and the patient's expectations for treatments
- details about the patient's lifestyle, family relationships, and cultural influences (during discharge planning, you'll need information about the patient's living arrangements, caregivers, resources, and support systems).

CHART QUICK

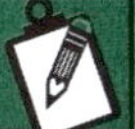

Integrated admission database form

Most health care facilities use a multidisciplinary admission form. The sample form below has spaces that can be filled in by the nurse, physician, and other health care providers.

Name *Beatrice Perry*
Address *2 Clayton Street*
Dallas, TX 55532
Admission date *6/27/02*
Time *1345*
Admitted per: ___ Ambulatory
✓ Stretcher ___ Wheelchair
T *97* P *92* R *24* BP *98/52*
Ht. *5'2"* Wt. *225 lb*
(estimated/actual)

Orientation to room/unit policies explained

✓ Call light
✓ Bed oper.
✓ Phone
✓ Television
✓ Meals
___ Advance directive explained
✓ Living will on chart
___ Valuables form completed
___ Elec.
✓ Smoking
✓ Side rails
___ ID bracelet on
✓ Visiting hours

Section completed by: *K. Crawford, CST* Time: *1350*

Name and phone numbers of two people to call if necessary:

Name	Relationship	Phone #
Mary Ryan	*daughter*	*665-2190*
John Carr	*son*	*665-4785*

Reason for hospitalization (patient quote:) *I go numb in my rt. arm and leg*
Anticipated date of discharge: *6/30/02*

Previous hospitalizations: Surgery/Illness	Date
TIA	*5/4/02*

FALL RISK /

Impaired:
___ sensory function
___ urinary/GI function
___ mobility function
___ mental status
___ general debility/weakness
✓ history of recent falls/dizziness/blackouts
✓ prone-to-fall risk (indicated on nursing Kardex ✓)

NEUROLOGICAL

___ Dizziness ___ Syncope ___ Headache ___ Blurred vision ___ Recent seizure
✓ Numbness/tingling location: *rt. arm and leg*

LOC:	✓ Alert	___ Lethargic	___ Semicomatose	___ Comatose
Mental Status:	✓ Oriented	___ Confused	___ Disoriented	
Speech:	✓ Clear	___ Slurred	___ Garbled	___ Aphasic

Neurological Checklist

Right Arm / Left arm	Right Leg / Left Leg	Right Pupil / Left Pupil	Pupil Reaction	Coma Scale: Eyes Open	Coma Scale: Best Verbal Response	Coma Scale: Best Motor Response	Coma Scale: Total
+2/+4	*+2/+4*	*5/6*	*+*	*4*	*5*	*6*	*15*

Pupil reaction
- Reactive
- Nonreactive
D Dilated
C Constricted
> Greater than
< Less than
? Equal
? Sluggish

CODE
Pupils: mm
1 2 3 4 5 6 7

(continued)

Integrated admission database form *(continued)*

PULMONARY

Respirations: √ Regular ___ Irregular
___ Shortness of breath ___ Dyspnea on exertion
O_2 use at home? ___ Yes √ No
Chest expansion: √ Symmetrical ___ Asymmetrical (explain): ___
Breath sounds: ___ Clear ___ Crackles ___ Rhonchi √ Wheezing
Location *bilat upper lobe, inspiratory*
Cough: √ None ___ Nonproductive ___ Productive
Describe ___
Comments: *pulse oximetry 98% on 2 Li sleeps with 2 pillows*

GASTROINTESTINAL

Stool: √ Formed
___ Loose
___ Liquid
___ Mucus
___ Ostomy
___ Incontinent

Color: √ Brown
___ Black
___ Red tinged
___ Bloody

Diarrhea ___
Constipation ___
Abdomen: √ Soft
___ Rigid
√ Nontender
___ Tender
___ (Location)
Bowel Sounds: √ Present
___ Absent
___ Hypoactive
___ Hyperactive

***Nutrition:**
√ Special Diet *1800 ADA*
___ Tube feeding
___ Chewing problem
___ Swallowing problems
___ Nausea/vomiting
___ Poor appetite
___ Wt. loss/gain ___ lb.

*refer to dietitian if any ✓

Obese √ Thin ___ Emaciated ___ Nourished ___

DISCHARGE PLANNING

Resources notified:	Name	Date	Time	Signature
Social worker				
Home care coordinator	*M. Murphy, RN*	*6/28/02*	*0900*	
Other				

Equipment/Supplies needed: *stair chair*
Arranged for by: *M. Murphy, RN* Date: *6/28/02* Time *0930*
Comment: *daughter to stay with pt at home*

DISCHARGE SUMMARY

Alterations in patterns: If yes, explain.	Yes	No	Explanation
Nutrition	√		*adherence to ADA diet regimen*
Elimination		√	
Self-care		√	
Skin integrity		√	
Mobility	√		*needs help with stairs*
Comfort pain		√	
Mental status/behavior		√	
Vision/Hearing/Speech		√	

Discharge instructions given (specify): *standard hosp. discharge instruction sheet*
Effects of illness on employment/lifestyle: ___
Central venous line removed: *N/A* By whom: ___
Belongings sent with patient: √ clothes √ dentures √ eyeglasses
___ hearing aid ___ prosthesis ___ valuables √ prescriptions √ other *cane*
Follow-up medical supervision to be provided by: *Dr. Schron*
√ Patient/family instructed to call for follow-up appointment
Discharge destination: *pt's home with daughter*
Section completed by: *C. Rafferty, RN* Date: *6/30/02* Time: *1215*

HOW TO USE THE ADMISSION DATABASE FORM

Conduct the patient interview and record the information on the admission form or progress notes as soon as possible, noting the date and time of the entry.

Acute illness, short hospital stays, and staff shortages can make it difficult to conduct a thorough and accurate initial interview. In some cases, you can ask the patient to complete a questionnaire about his past and present health status and you can use this to document his health history.

Before completing the admission database form, consider the patient's ability and readiness to participate. For example, if he's sedated, confused, hostile, angry, or having pain or breathing problems, ask only the most essential questions. You can perform an in-depth interview later, when his condition improves.

During your interview, try to alleviate as much of the patient's discomfort and anxiety as possible. Also, try to create a quiet, private environment for your talk.

If the patient can't provide information, consider seeking help from friends or family members. Be sure to document your sources. If the patient is too ill to be interviewed and family members aren't available, base your initial assessment on your observations and physical examination. Be sure to document on the admission form why you couldn't obtain complete data, and then obtain the rest of the information as soon as possible.

POTENTIAL PROBLEMS

Admission database forms can present some difficulties. At times, through no fault of your own, you won't be able to complete some forms. The quality of recorded data depends in part on the ability of the patient or members of his family to provide accurate information.

Many other people will document on the integrated admission database forms, increasing the risk of missing or incorrect information. You can't assume that colleagues collected the right information. You're responsible for verifying and correcting information gathered by nursing assistants and licensed practical nurses; likewise, the physician is responsible for verifying information that you've collected. Remember, adding new information later may require you to revise the care plan accordingly.

Care plans and critical pathways

In acute care settings today, two different formats are being used to guide the process of care for a patient:

- traditional care plan
- critical pathway.

Both formats offer important advantages and disadvantages. The traditional care plan, based on a nursing assessment and nursing diagnosis, provides a more precise account of the patient's individual nursing needs. The standardized critical pathway is a better tool for facilitating interdisciplinary communication and is perhaps more suited to the demands of the managed care environment.

CARE PLANS

The full nursing care needs of any patient are unlikely to be documented on a critical pathway. For this reason, some acute care facilities are continuing to rely on the traditional format of a care plan as the chief mechanism for documenting each patient's nursing care.

Although JCAHO no longer requires a specific care-planning format, the commission does require that the following information be included in care plans in an acute care setting:

- ongoing assessments of the patient's illness and response to care, including patient needs, concerns, problems, capabilities, and limitations
- ongoing evaluation and modification of nursing diagnoses, interventions, and expected outcomes, based on identified patient needs and care priorities
- notation of nursing interventions, patient monitoring and surveillance, and patient responses
- reevaluation of patient progress compared with goals and the care plan
- documentation of the inability to meet patient care goals and the reason for this.

CRITICAL PATHWAYS

Many acute care facilities are abandoning the traditional care plan in favor of a standardized critical pathway. Critical pathways are combinations of multidisciplinary care plans.

The changeover from plan to pathway has thrown nursing documentation into a transitional state. You may find yourself working in a facility that uses both formats. Many nurses aren't yet comfortable with critical pathways and are double-documenting—copying information from a pathway into a care plan.

Critical pathways are used in health care facilities that employ case management systems for delivering care. In such a system, a registered nurse acting as case manager oversees a closely monitored and controlled system of multidisciplinary care.

Nurses, physicians, and other health care providers are responsible for establishing a care track, or case map, for each diagnosis-related group (DRG). A DRG is a way of classifying a patient according to his medical diagnosis for the purpose of obtaining reimbursement for facility costs. The care track is used to determine a patient's daily care requirements and desired outcomes. The average length of stay for the patient's DRG is used in defining the care track. The case manager oversees achievement of outcomes, length of stay, and the use of equipment throughout the patient's illness.

For acute care facilities, critical pathways work best with diagnoses that have fairly predictable outcomes—for example, hip replacement, cerebrovascular accident, myocardial infarction, or open heart surgery. The pathway is a way to standardize and organize care for routine conditions. It makes it easier for the case manager to track data needed to streamline use of materials and human resources, ensure that patients receive quality care, improve coordination of care, and reduce the cost of care.

Health care facilities have a financial incentive to switch to critical pathway documentation. Well-developed critical pathways with demonstrated cost reductions may provide the facility with an advantage when negotiating contracts with managed care organizations.

Using a critical pathway doesn't eliminate the need for nurses to diagnose and treat human responses to health problems. Patients are individuals and commonly require nursing intervention beyond that specified in the critical pathway.

For example, a patient enters the facility for a hip replacement and can't communicate verbally because of a previous stroke. The critical pathway wouldn't include measures to assist this patient in making his needs known. Therefore, you would develop a nursing care plan around the nursing diagnosis *Impaired verbal communication*. By using the critical pathway and developing a nursing care plan based on the patient's individual nursing diagnoses, you can provide the best in collaborative care.

Patient care Kardex

The patient care Kardex, sometimes called the nursing Kardex, gives a quick overview of basic patient care information. A Kardex can be computer generated, or it may be on a large index card that typically contains boxes that allow you to check off items that apply to each patient. It also contains space for recording current orders for medications, patient care activities, treatments, and tests. (See *Components of a patient care Kardex,* pages 100 and 101.)

A Kardex isn't a JCAHO requirement. Some facilities have eliminated Kardexes, incorporating the information they contain into the patient's care plan.

Refer to the Kardex during change-of-shift reports and throughout the day. The information it contains includes:

- patient's name, age, marital status, and religion
- medical diagnoses, listed by priority
- nursing diagnoses, listed by priority
- current doctors' orders for medication, treatments, diet, I.V. therapy, diagnostic tests, procedures, and other measures
- consultations
- results of diagnostic tests and procedures
- permitted activities, functional limitations, assistance that's needed, and safety precautions.

Kardexes come in various shapes, sizes, and types and may be computer generated. Some facilities use different Kardexes to document specific information, such as medication information, test results, and nonnursing data.

Typically used to record laboratory or diagnostic test results and X-ray findings, a computerized Kardex usually includes information on medical orders, referrals, consultations, specimens (for culture and sensitivity tests or for blood glucose analysis, for example), vital signs, diet, and activity restrictions. (See *Computer-generated patient care Kardex,* page 102.)

ADVANTAGES

The Kardex has some good points, including the following:

- It allows quick access to information about task-oriented interventions, such as specific patient care, medication administration, and I.V. therapy.
- The care plan may be added to the Kardex to provide all the necessary

CHART QUICK

Components of a patient care Kardex

Here's an example of a patient care Kardex for a medical-surgical unit. Its brief phrases are intended to trigger images of procedures, activities, or patient conditions. A Kardex for a critical care, obstetric, or other unit has additional unit-specific topics (see middle and lower sections on page 101).

Care status
- Self-care ☐
- Partial care with assistance ☐
- Complete care ☑
- Shower with assistance ☑
- Tub ☐
- Active exercises ☐
- Passive exercises ☐

Special care
- Back care ☑
- Mouth care ☑
- Foot care ☐
- Perineal care ☑
- Catheter care ☐
- Tracheostomy care ☐
- Other (specify)________ ☐

Condition
- Satisfactory ☐
- Fair ☐
- Guarded ☑
- Critical ☐
- No code ☐
- Advance directive?
  - Yes ☑
  - No ☐
- Date *5/12/02*

Prosthesis
- Dentures
  - upper ☑
  - lower ☑
- Contact lenses ☐
- Glasses ☑
- Hearing aid ☑
- Other (specify)________ ☐

Isolation
- Strict ☐
- Contact ☐
- Airborne ☑
- Neutropenic ☐
- Droplet ☐
- Other (specify)________ ☐

Diet
- Type: *low-fat, no conc. sweets*
- Force fluids ☐
- NPO ☐
- Assist with feeding ☐
- Isolation tray ☑
- Calorie count ☐
- Supplements ____________

Tube feedings ☐
- Type: ____________
- Rate: ____________
- Route: ____________
  - NG ☐
  - G tube ☐
  - J tube ☐

Admission
- Height: *60"*
- Weight *145 lb (67 kg)*
- BP: *124/72*
- TPR: *100.4 T P.O. – 92–24*

Frequency
- BP: *q shift*
- TPR: *q shift*
- Apical pulses:
- Peripheral pulses: *q shift*
- Weight:
- Neuro check:
- Monitor:
- Strips:
- Turn:
- Cough: *q shift*
- Deep breathe: *q shift*
- Central venous pressure:
- Other (specify)________

GI tubes
- Salem sump ☐
- Levin tube ☐
- Feeding tube ☐
- Type (specify)________
- Other (specify)________ ☐

Activity
- Bed rest ☐
- Chair t.i.d. ☑
- Dangle ☐
- Commode ☐
- Commode with assist ☑
- Ambulate ☑
- BRP ☑
- Fall-risk category (specify):________ ☐
- Other (specify)________ ☐

Mode of transport
- Wheelchair ☑
- Stretcher ☐
- With oxygen ☐

I.V. devices
- Saline lock ☐
- Peripheral I.V. ☐
- Central line ☑
- Triple-lumen CVP ☐
- Hickman ☐
- Jugular ☐
- Peripherally inserted ☐
- PICC ☐
- Parenteral nutrition ☐
- Irrigations ____________

Dressings
- Type: *CVP*
- Change: *as needed*

Components of a patient care Kardex *(continued)*

Respiratory therapy
Pulse oximetry: ________
SVO_2 level (%): ________
Oxygen ☑
Liters/min. 2 L/minute ☑
Method
- Nasal cannula ☑
- Face mask ☐
- Venturi (Venti) mask ☐
- Nonrebreather mask ☐
- Trach collar ☐

Nebulizer ☑
Chest PT ☐
Incentive spirometry ☑
T-piece ☐
Ventilator ☐
- Type: ________
- Settings: ________

Other (specify) ________ ☐

Drains
Type: ________
Number: ________
Location: ________

Urine output
I&O ☑
Strain urine ☐
Indwelling catheter ☐
- Date inserted ________
- Size: ________

Intermittent catheter ☐
- Frequency: ________

Side rails
Constant ☐
PRN ☐
Nights ☐

Restraints
Date: ________
Type: ________

Specimens and tests
CBC daily
24-hour collection
Other (specify) ________

Stools

Special notes

Social services
Consulted 5/12/02

Monitoring
Hardwire ☑
Telemetry ☐

Pulmonary artery catheter ☑
- Pulmonary artery pressure ________
- Pulmonary artery wedge pressure ________

CVP ☐
Arterial line ☐
Other (specify) ICP ☑

Mechanical ventilation
Type: ________
Tidal volume: ________
FIO_2: ________
Mode: ________
Rate: ________

Delivery
Date: 5/4/02
Time: 0725
Type of delivery: c-section

Special procedures
Perineal rinse ☐
Sitz bath ☐
Witch hazel compress ☐
Breast binders ☐
Ice ☐
Abdominal binders ☑
Other (specify) ________ ☐

Mother
Due date: ________
Gravida: ________
Para: ________
Rh: ________
Blood type: ________
Membranes ruptured: ________
Episiotomy ☐
Lacerations ☐
RhoGAM studies?
- Yes ☐
- No ☐

Rubella titer?
- Yes ☐
- No ☐

Infant
Male ☐
Female ☐
Full-term ☐
Premature ☐
- Weeks ☐

Apgar score ☐
Nursing ☐
Formula ☐
Condition (specify) ________
Other (specify) ________

CHART QUICK

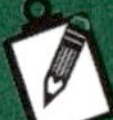

Computer-generated patient care Kardex

In the computer-generated Kardex shown below, you'll find a detailed list of medical orders and other patient care data.

6/11/02 1359 PAGE 001

Jones, John M 73
MR#: 000310593 acct#: 9400037290
DR: J. Becher 2/W 204-01
Dx: Exacerbation COPD DATE: 6/11/02

SUMMARY: 6/11 0701 to 1501

PATIENT INFORMATION

6/11	ADVANCE DIRECTIVE: Yes
6/11	ORGAN DONOR: Yes
6/11	ADMIT Dx: Exacerbation COPD
6/11	MED ALLERGY: PCN
6/11	ISOLATION: Standard precautions

MISC. PATIENT DATA

NURSING CARE PLAN PROBLEMS:

6/11 Ineffective breathing pattern R/T fatigue

ALL CURRENT MEDICAL ORDERS

NURSING ORDERS:

6/11	Activity, OOB, Up as tolerated
6/11	Routine V/S q8h
6/11	Telemetry
6/11	If 0700 pulse OX > 93%, decrease O_2 to 1 L nasal cannula

DIET:

6/11 2 g Na

IVS:

6/11 Peripheral line #1....Start aminophylline 1 g in 250 D_5W: rate, 35 mg/hour

data for patient care, although this duplicates information.

DISADVANTAGES

The Kardex has one major drawback: It's only as useful as nurses make it. It isn't an effective documenting tool if there isn't enough space for appropriate information, if it isn't updated frequently, if it isn't completed, or if it isn't read before giving patient care.

In addition, Kardexes aren't usually part of the permanent record, so make sure the information on the Kardex is also found elsewhere on the patient's chart.

HOW TO USE THE KARDEX

The Kardex is most effective when you tailor the information to the needs of a particular setting. For instance, an intensive care unit Kardex should include information on hardwire or telemetry monitoring and arterial pressure monitoring.

Use the Kardex to record information that helps nurses plan daily interventions. For example, record the time a patient prefers to bathe, his food preferences before and during chemotherapy, and which analgesics or positions are usually required to ease pain.

The medication Kardex

If your facility uses a separate medication Kardex on acute care units, you'll find this document on the medication cart or other designated place. The medication Kardex may include the medication administration record (MAR), which lists medications, doses, and frequency and route of administration. Medication administration is documented on this form, which is a permanent part of the patient's record. (See *The medication Kardex,* pages 104 and 105.)

Here are some tips for recording information on a medication Kardex:

- Include the date and administration time as well as the medication dose, route, and frequency. Don't forget to initial the entry.
- Indicate when you administer a *stat* dose of a medication and, if appropriate, the number of doses ordered and the stop date.
- Write legibly, using only standard abbreviations. When in doubt about how to abbreviate a term, spell it out. Remember, the MAR is a legal record, so any information entered there should be legible and above question.
- After giving the first dose of a medication, sign your full name, your licensure status, and your initials in the appropriate space.
- After withholding a medication dose, document which dose wasn't given (usually by circling the time it was scheduled). Also document the reason it was omitted (for example, withholding oral medications from a patient because he has surgery scheduled that day).

If you administer all medications according to the care plan, you don't need to document further. However, if your MAR doesn't have space for some information — such as the parenteral administration site, the patient's response to as-needed medications, or deviations from the medication order — you'll need to record this information in the progress notes. For example, you need to document the reason you don't administer a medication such as *Digoxin held per order of Dr. John because of pt's heart rate of 53. Digoxin level pending.*

Graphic form

The graphic form is used to plot the patient's vital signs. Weight, intake and output, appetite, and activity level also may be documented on the graphic form. (See *Using a graphic form,* page 106.)

The graphic form usually has a column of data printed on the left side of the page, times and dates written across the top, and open blocks within the side and top borders.

(Text continues on page 106.)

CHART QUICK

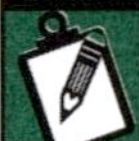

The medication Kardex

One type of Kardex is the medication Kardex. It contains a permanent record of the patient's medications. The medication Kardex may also include the patient's diagnosis and information about allergies and diet. A sample form is shown here.

Nurse's full signature, status, and initials

	Init.		Init.		Init.
Roy Charles, RN	RC				
Theresa Hopkins, RN	TH				

Diagnoses: Heart failure, Atrial flutter

Allergies: ASA | Diet: Cardiac

Routine/daily orders/finger sticks/insulin coverage				Date: 6/24/02		Date:	
Order date / Init.	Renewal date / Init.	Medications dose, route, frequency	Time	Site	Init.	Site	Init.
6/24/02		digoxin 0.125 mg	0900	(R) s.c.	RC		
RC		I.V. q.d.	HR	76			
6/24/02		furosemide 40 mg	0900	(R) s.c.	RC		
RC		I.V. q 12h	2100	(R) s.c.	TH		
6/24/02		enalapril	1100	(R) s.c.	TH		
RC		1.25 mg I.V. q6h	1700	(R) s.c.	RC		
6/25/02		vancomycin 1 g I.V. q.d.	2100	(R) s.c.	TH		
TH							

The medication Kardex *(continued)*

Addressograph				PRN medication Allergies: ASA			
Init.	Signature and status	Init.	Signature and status	Init.	Signature and status	Init.	Signature and status
RC	Roy Charles, RN						
TH	Theresa Hopkins, RN						

Year 20 02 — P.R.N. medications

Order						
Order Date: 6/24 · Renewal Date: · Discontinued Date:		Date	6/24		
Medication: acetaminophen	Dose 650 mg	Time given	0930		
Direction: p.r.n. mild pain	Route P.O.	Data			
		Init.	RC		
Order Date: 6/24 · Renewal Date: · Discontinued Date:		Date	6/24		
Medication: MSO_4	Dose 2 mg	Time given	0930		
Direction: 15 minutes prior to changing Ⓡ heel dressing	Route I.V.	Data			
		Init.	RC		
Order Date: 6/24 · Renewal Date: · Discontinued Date:		Date	6/24		
Medication: Milk of Magnesia	Dose 30 ml	Time given	2115		
Direction: q 6h p.r.n	Route P.O.	Data			
		Init.	TH		
Order Date: 6/25 · Renewal Date: · Discontinued Date:		Date	6/25		
Medication: prochlorperazine	Dose 5 mg	Time given	1100	2230	
Direction: q 8h p.r.n. p.r.n. nausea and vomiting	Route I.M.	Data P.O.	Ⓡ glut	Ⓛ glut	
		Init.	RC	TH	
Order Date: · Renewal Date: · Discontinued Date:		Date			
Medication:	Dose	Time given			
Direction:	Route	Data			
		Init.			
Order Date: · Renewal Date: · Discontinued Date:		Date			
Medication:	Dose	Time given			
Direction:	Route	Data			
		Init.			

CHART QUICK

Using a graphic form

Plotting information on a graphic form helps you visualize changes in your patient's temperature, blood pressure, heart rate, weight, and intake and output. Review the sample form below.

GRAPHIC FORM

Instructions: Indicate temp. in "0" and pulse in"X"

Date Hosp. day	7/1/02 3			
Postop. day	2			

	4	8	12	4	8	12	4	8	12	4	8	12	4	8	12	4	8	12	4	8	12	4	8	12
Pulse F																								
150 106°																								
140 105°																								
130 104°																								
120 103°																								
110 102°																								
100 101°																								
90 100°																								
80 99°																								
70 98°																								
60 97°																								
50 96°																								
95°																								
Respiration		18			22																			

Blood pressure	120/80 138/80			

INTAKE	7-3	3-11	11-7	7-3	3-11	11-7	7-3	3-11	11-7	7-3	3-11	11-7
P.O.	480	800	600									
I.V.		100	100									
Blood/Colloid	250	900	0									
8-hour	730	1800	700									
24-hour	3230											
OUTPUT	7-3	3-11	11-7	7-3	3-11	11-7	7-3	3-11	11-7	7-3	3-11	11-7
Urine	800	550	500									
NG/Emesis	0	50	0									
Other	0	0	0									
8-hour	800	600	500									
24-hour	1900											
Weight	150 lb											
Stool	0	0	+									

ADVANTAGES

The graphic form has two important advantages:

- It presents information at a glance. This allows more visual comparison of data than is possible in narrative-style forms. For example, if a patient's temperature goes up or down or fluctuates over time, this can be detected much more readily on a graph than in a narrative account of the patient's temperature.

- Unlicensed personnel, such as nursing assistants and technicians, are allowed to document measurements on graphic forms, saving nurses valuable time.

DISADVANTAGES

Graphic forms also have the following disadvantages:

- If data placed on the graph aren't accurate, legible, and complete, the form is useless. Every vital sign you take should be transcribed onto the form. For accuracy, double-check the graph after transcribing information.
- If you use information from the graph alone, you won't get a complete picture of the patient's clinical condition. You must combine the graph with narrative documentation.

HOW TO USE A GRAPHIC FORM

To avoid transcription errors, document directly onto a graphic form when information is obtained.

If a medication (an antipyretic or antihypertensive, for example) precipitates a change in a particular vital sign, document this in the progress notes as well as on the graphic form. Specify the relationship between the medication and its effect.

Make sure you also document vital signs on both the graphic form and the progress notes when a patient has an acute episode, such as chest pain or a seizure. Be sure to:

- document legibly
- put data in the correct time line
- make the dots you plot on the graph large enough to be seen easily (connect the dots if your facility requires this).

Progress notes and flow sheets

In the acute care setting, progress notes and flow sheets are used to record the patient's status and monitor changes in his condition.

PROGRESS NOTES

Progress notes are written chronologically. The standard format for nursing progress notes has a column for the date and time and a column for detailed comments about:

- the patient's problems (the nursing diagnoses)
- the patient's needs
- pertinent nursing observations
- nursing reassessments and interventions
- the patient's responses to interventions
- evaluation of expected outcomes.

All members of the health care team can document integrated progress notes, which are in chronological order based on the date. (See *Integrated progress notes*, page 108.)

Advantages

Progress notes are helpful for the following reasons:

- They're written chronologically and reflect the nursing diagnoses.
- They contain narrative information that doesn't easily fit into available space or format provided by other documentation forms.

CHART QUICK

Integrated progress notes

One key advantage of integrated progress notes: Every member of the health care team can document on them. Integrated progress notes are written in chronological order and dated.

INTEGRATED PROGRESS NOTES

6/24/02 0800 Nursing note
Pt with temp. 102° F. Doctor Weber notified. No order at this time. — P. Smith, RN
6/24/02 0830 MICU attending
Pt continues to appear w/o change in status. Remains febrile and unresponsive. Will discuss code status with family. Prognosis poor. — R. Weber, MD
6/24/02 1030 Infectious disease attending
Pt continues with fever of unknown origin. T max. 104° F. Tylenol ineffective. Cultures from 6/23 pending. Change all central line accesses and send tips for culture. Continue vancomycin, gentamicin, and amikacin. Monitor trough levels and adjust dosages accordingly. Try to obtain HIV testing consent from family. Send fungal cultures. If positive for fungemia, amphotericin B. Use test dose. Consult renal for worsening renal failure — J. Barry, MD
6/24/02 1545 Intern progress note
HIV consent obtained. Labs to be drawn. — J. Krimm, DO

Disadvantages

On the other hand, progress notes have these pitfalls:

- If they aren't well organized, you may have to read through the entire form to find what you're looking for. To help prevent this, some facilities require you to put a heading on each note.
- You may waste time recording information on progress notes that you have already recorded on other forms.

How to write progress notes

When writing progress notes, include the following information:

- date and time of the entry
- the patient's condition
- interventions
- the patient's response to care
- details of changes in the patient's condition
- evaluation of interventions.

Some progress notes are designed to focus on nursing diagnoses. If your facility uses this type of note, be sure to record the nursing diagnosis that relates to your entry.

Every time you write a progress note, be sure to record the exact time you gave the care or noted the observation. Don't record entries in blocks of time, such as *3:30 to 8:30.* Years ago, when nurses were required to write progress notes every 2 hours, documenting blocks of time was common. But today, most nurses use a flow sheet to document how often they check on a patient. Together, flow sheets and progress notes usually provide adequate evidence of nursing care.

Be sure to document new patient problems, such as *Onset of seizures,* and the resolution of old problems, such as *No complaint of pain in 12 hours*. Also, record deteriorations in the patient's condition — for example, *Pt has increasing dyspnea, causing him to remain on bed rest. ABG values show* Pao_2 *of 55.* O_2 *provided by rebreather mask as ordered.*

Document your observations of the patient's response to the care plan. If his behaviors are similar to agreed-upon objectives, document that the goals are being met. If not, document that they aren't being met.

Avoid including information that's already on the flow sheet, except when there's a sudden change in the patient's condition, such as a decreased level of consciousness, a change in skin condition, or swelling at an I.V. site.

Sometimes, nurses document a problem but fail to describe what they did about it. Outline your interventions clearly, including such information as notification of other health team members, interventions, and the patient's response. For example, *Pt at 8 a.m. had oral temp of 102° F, Dr. Bard notified. Acetaminophen 650 mg given P.O. At 10 a.m. pt had oral temp of 100° F.*

Avoid vague wording. Using a phrase like "appears to be" indicates uncertainty about what you're documenting. Phrases like "no problems" and "had a good day" are also ambiguous. Document specific observations instead. For example, *Pt reports his left hip has less pain, a 2 on a scale of 1 to 10. Yesterday it was a 5.*

FLOW SHEETS

Flow sheets highlight specific patient information according to preestablished parameters of nursing care. They have spaces for recording dates, times, and specific interventions, which are set by each facility.

Flow sheets are used for documenting data related to physical assessment of the patient and for recording routine aspects of patient care, such as activities of daily living, fluid balance, nutrition, pain, and skin integrity. They're also useful for recording specific nursing interventions.

Many facilities also document I.V. therapy and patient education on flow sheets. The style and format of flow sheets may vary to fit the needs of patients on particular units. Using flow sheets doesn't exempt you from narrative charting to describe your observations, patient teaching, patient responses, detailed interventions, and unusual circumstances. (See *Using flow sheets to document routine care*, pages 110 and 111.)

Advantages

Flow sheets offer many advantages:

- You can insert nursing data quickly and concisely, preferably at the time you give care or observe a change in the patient's condition.
- Because they provide an easy-to-read record of changes in the patient's condition over time, flow sheets allow all members of the health care team to compare data and assess the patient's progress.
- The concise format enables you to evaluate patient trends at a glance.
- They're less time consuming to read because they tend to be more legible than handwritten progress notes.

CHART QUICK

Using flow sheets to document routine care

As this sample shows, a patient care flow sheet lets you quickly document routine interventions.

PATIENT CARE FLOW SHEET

Date: 6/22/02	2300-0700	0700-1500	1500-2300
Respiratory			
Breath sounds	Clear 2330 AS	Crackles LLL 0800 JM	Clear 1600 HM
Treatments/ Results	———	Nebulizer 0830 JM	———
Cough/ Results	———	Mod. amt. tenacious yellow mucus 0900 JM	———
O_2 therapy	Nasal cannula @2 L/min AS	Nasal cannula @2 L/min JM	Nasal cannula @2 L/min HM
Cardiac			
Chest pain	———	———	———
Heart sounds	Normal S_1 and S_2 AS	Normal S_1 and S_2 JM	Normal S_1 and S_2 HM
Telemetry	N/A	N/A	N/A
Pain			
Type and location	Ⓛ flank 0400 AS	Ⓛ flank 1000 JM	Ⓛ flank 1600 HM
Intervention	meperidine 0415 AS	reposition and meperidine 1010 JM	meperidine 1615 HM
Pt response	Improved from #9 to #3 in 1/2 hour AS	Improved from #8 to #2 in 1/2 hr JM	Complete relief in 1 hr HM
Nutrition			
Type	———	regular JM	Regular HM
Toleration %	———	90% JM	80% HM
Supplement	———	1 can Ensure JM	———
Elimination			
Stool appearance	———	———	———
Enema	N/A	N/A	N/A
Results	———	———	———
Bowel sounds	present all quadrants 2330 AS	present all quadrants 0800 JM	hyperactive all quadrants 1600 HM
Urine appearance	Clear amber 0400 AS	Clear amber 1000 JM	Dark yellow 1500 HM
Indwelling urinary catheter	N/A	N/A	N/A
Catheter irrigations	———	———	———

Using flow sheets to document routine care *(continued)*

PATIENT CARE FLOW SHEET

Date: 6/22/02	2300-0700	0700-1500	1500-2300
Tubes			
Type	N/A	N/A	N/A
Irrigation	—	—	—
Drainage appearance	—	—	—
Hygiene			
Self/partial/ complete	—	Partial 1000 JM	Partial 2100 HM
Oral care	—	1000 JM	2100 HM
Back care	0400 AS	1000 JM	2100 HM
Foot care	—	1000 JM	—
Remove/ reapply elastic stockings	2330 AS	1000 JM	2100 HM
Activity			
Type	bed rest AS	OOB to chair x 20 min 1000 JM	OOB to chair x 20 min 1800 HM
Toleration	Turns self AS	Tol. well JM	Tol. well HM
Repositioned	2330 supine AS 0400 Ⓛ side AS	Ⓛ side 0800 JM Ⓡ side 1400 JM	self HM
ROM	—	1000 (active) JM 1400 (active) JM	1800 (active) HM 2200 (active) HM
Sleep			
Sleeps well	0400 AS 0600 AS	N/A	N/A
Awake at intervals	2300 AS 0400 AS	—	—
Awake most of the time	—	—	—
Safety			
ID bracelet on	2330 AS 0200 AS	0800 JM 1200 JM 1500 JM	1600 HM 2100 HM
Call button in reach	2330 AS 0200 AS	0800 JM 1200 JM 1500 JM	1600 HM 2100 HM
Side rails up	2330 AS 0200 AS	0800 JM 1200 JM 1500 JM	1600 HM 2100 HM

- The format reinforces standards of nursing care and facilitates precise and less fragmented nursing documentation.

Disadvantages

Flow sheets also have some drawbacks:

- They may not have enough space for recording unusual events.

- Overuse of these forms can lead to incomplete documentation that obscures the patient's clinical picture.
- They may cause legal hassles if they aren't consistent with the progress notes. What's checked off on the flow sheet needs to agree with what's documented on the progress notes.
- The format may fail to reflect the patients' needs as well as the nurses' documentation needs on each unit. Flow sheets can become a liability if they aren't tailored to each unit and revised as needed.

How to use flow sheets

Ideally, flow sheets are used to document all routine assessment data and nursing interventions. Some common examples of these are:

- repositioning or turning the patient
- range-of-motion exercises
- patient education
- wound care
- medication administration.

Documenting routine assessment data this way allows you to focus on changes in the patient's condition, his complex needs, and his progress toward achieving expected outcomes. Make sure that data on the flow sheet are consistent with data in your progress notes. Of course, all entries should accurately reflect the care given. Discrepancies can damage your credibility and increase your chance of liability.

Sometimes, recording only the information requested isn't enough to give a complete picture of the patient's health. If this is the case, record additional information in the space provided on the flow sheet. If additional information isn't necessary, draw a line through the space to indicate this.

If your flow sheet doesn't have additional space and you need to record more information, use the progress notes.

Fill out flow sheets completely, using the specified symbols — such as check marks, "X"s, initials, circles, or the time — to indicate assessment of a parameter or performance of an intervention. When necessary, use the abbreviation "N/A" (not applicable) or another abbreviation recognized by your facility.

Don't leave blank spaces, which may imply that an intervention wasn't completed, wasn't attempted, or wasn't recognized. If you must omit something, document the reason for the omission.

Discharge summaries

Discharge summaries reflect the reassessment and evaluation components of the nursing process. To comply with JCAHO requirements, you must document your assessment of a patient's continuing care needs as well as any referrals for care and begin discharge planning early in the patient's stay.

To help in this kind of documentation, many facilities combine discharge summaries and patient instructions in one form. This form contains sections for recording patient assessment, patient education, detailed special instructions, and the circumstances of discharge. It uses a narrative style along with open- and closed-ended styles. (See *Using discharge summaries.*)

CHART QUICK

Using discharge summaries

By combining the patient's discharge summary with instructions for care after discharge, you can fulfill two requirements with a single form. When using this documentation method, be sure to give one copy to the patient and keep one for the record.

DISCHARGE INSTRUCTIONS

1. Summary Tara Nicholas is a 55 year old woman admitted with complaints of severe headache and hypertensive crisis.
Treatment: Nipride gtt for 24 hours
Started Lopressor for hypertension
Recommendation: Lose 10–15 lbs
Follow low Na, low cholesterol diet

2. Allergies penicillin
3. Medications (drug, dose time) Lopressor 25 mg at 6am and 6pm
temazepam 15 mg at 10pm
4. Diet Low sodium, low cholesterol
5. Activity As tolerated
6. Discharged to Home
7. If questions arise, contact Dr. Pritchett Telephone no. 525-1448
8. Special instructions
9. Return visit Dr. Pritchett Place Health Care Clinic
On date 6/15/02 Time 8:45 am

Tara Nicholas — Signature of patient for receipt of instructions from doctors

JE Pritchett MD — Signature of physician giving instructions

ADVANTAGES

Discharge summary forms have no disadvantages, only benefits:

- The combined form provides useful data about additional teaching needs and points out whether the patient has the information he needs to care for himself or to get further help.
- The form establishes compliance with JCAHO requirements and helps safeguard you from malpractice accusations.

HOW TO USE DISCHARGE SUMMARIES

After completing your discharge summary form, give one copy to the patient and put another copy in the medical record for future reference. Make sure the completed form outlines the patient's care, provides useful information for further teaching and evaluation, and documents that the patient has the information he needs to care for himself or to get further help.

Not all facilities use combined forms — some use narrative discharge

CHART QUICK

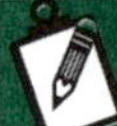

Narrative discharge notes

Some health care facilities use a narrative-style discharge summary, which is similar to a progress note. Here's a sample:

Date	Time	Progress notes
7/1/02	Discharge	68 y.o. black male admitted 6/28/02 with chest pain,
	1530	hypertension; BP 190/100, and SOB. MI ruled out. Chest
	(summary)	pain relieved with sublingual nitroglycerin and O_2.
		Persantine thallium performed 6/30. Tolerated proce-
		dure well. Has been OOB ambulating in the hallway with-
		out chest pain or SOB since 6/30. BP remains stable
		(144/86 at 1215). Drug regimen includes daily aspirin
		325 mg, and captopril 25 mg b.i.d. Verbalized under-
		standing of medication times, dosages, and adverse
		effects. Will call Dr. Harris for 10 day postdischarge
		appointment. Discharge instruction sheet given.
		B. McCort, RN

notes. (See *Narrative discharge notes.*) If your facility uses these, be sure to include the following information on the form:

- the patient's status at admission and discharge
- significant information about the patient's stay in the facility, including resolved and unresolved patient problems and referrals for continuing care
- instructions given to the patient, members of his family, and other caregivers about medications, treatments, activity, diet, referrals, follow-up appointments, and any other special instructions.

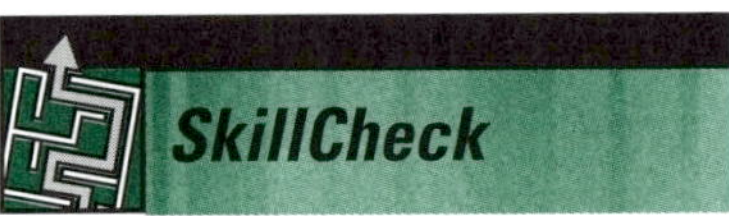

SkillCheck

1. Which documentation tool allows you to quickly compare data?

a. Protocol
b. Focus sheet
c. Initial assessment form
d. Flow sheet

Answer: d. Because they provide an easy-to-read record of changes in the patient's condition over time, flow sheets allow all members of the health care team to compare data.

2. What form should you use to document your initial patient assessment?

a. Nursing care plan
b. Progress notes
c. Admission assessment form
d. Kardex

Answer: c. The admission assessment form, also known as the admission database form, is used to document the broad scope of information usually obtained during the initial assessment.

3. Which of the following is true about the patient care Kardex?

a. It isn't usually part of the permanent record.
b. It's where you document a narrative note.
c. You don't have to update it frequently.
d. Every facility uses the same Kardex form.

Answer: a. Because it isn't usually part of the permanent record, make sure that the information on the Kardex can be found somewhere else in the patient's chart.

4. What is a major advantage of a discharge summary form?

a. Every facility uses one.
b. It doesn't include an area to document special instructions for patients.
c. It can help safeguard you from malpractice accusations.
d. It's where you document your interventions.

Answer: c. Discharge summaries can help safeguard you by complying with JCAHO requirements to include your assessment of a patient's continuing care needs and referrals for care in your documentation.

5. Progress notes are organized according to what order?

a. Alphabetical
b. Chronological
c. Numerical
d. The order you prefer

Answer: b. Progress notes chronologically record the patient's status and track changes in his condition.

5 Documenting in long-term care

A long-term care facility provides continuing care for the chronically ill or disabled patient. The purpose of care is to promote the highest level of functioning possible for the patient. Long-term care is an increasingly important form of health care delivery, especially because the elderly segment of the population is rapidly growing.

Maintaining accurate, complete documentation in long-term care is vital. Consider the following points:

- Long-term care facilities are highly regulated by state and federal agencies and therefore must live up to high standards of documentation.
- Information in your records may be used to defend you and your facility in court.
- Your employer views documentation records as evidence of standardized, high-quality nursing care.
- Good record keeping ensures certification, licensure, reimbursement, and accreditation.

Two key differences exist between documenting in long-term care settings and documenting in other settings:

- First, patients stay at long-term care facilities for weeks or months, so documentation isn't done as often. This takes the emphasis off documenting and puts it on helping the patient relearn basic skills.
- Second, some of the government forms used in long-term care facilities are long and involved. So even though documenting isn't emphasized, it can still be extensive.

Long-term care facilities usually offer two levels of care: skilled and intermediate. The level of care administered to your patient should be your primary consideration when documenting.

In a skilled care facility, patient care involves specialized nursing skills, such as I.V. therapy, parenteral nutrition, respiratory care, and mechanical ventilation.

An intermediate care facility deals with patients who have chronic illnesses and need less complex care. For example, they may simply need assistance with activities of daily living (ADLs), such as bathing and dressing.

Patients at both levels may need short- or long-term care and may move from one level to another according to their progress or decline. Living arrangements, geography, family and community support networks, and other factors determine the patient's length of stay.

Regulatory agencies

Documentation in long-term care facilities is regulated by federal and state agencies. Documentation is influenced by:

- federal programs, such as Medicare and Medicaid
- government agencies such as the Centers for Medicare & Medicaid Services (CMS)
- laws such as the Omnibus Budget Reconciliation Act (OBRA) of 1987
- state regulations for each facility
- accrediting agencies such as the Joint Commission on Accreditation of Healthcare Organizations (JCAHO).

Most elderly patients entering a long-term care facility pay for the services privately. If they exhaust their funds, they apply to Medicaid for coverage. The patient who requires services and can't pay initially may apply to receive Medicaid.

MEDICARE

Few of the services provided in long-term care facilities are eligible for Medicare reimbursement. However, Medicare does provide reimbursement for patients requiring skilled care, such as chemotherapy or tube feeding. For these patients, Medicare requires certain minimum daily documentation to prove that a service was needed. If the patient's status changes, you must supply a revised care plan within 7 days.

Be sure to document changes in status because a patient who isn't improving or isn't expected to improve according to his care plan is ineligible for coverage. You must also document the need for new or continuing skilled services you provide. Medicare also requires documentation of your evaluations for expected outcomes.

According to Medicare guidelines, documentation must clearly show that a patient needed care by a professional or technical staff member. To verify the need for skilled rehabilitative care, you must describe a reasonable expectation of improvement or services needed to establish a maintenance program. The amount, duration, and frequency of services must be reasonable and necessary.

MEDICAID

Most patients who receive skilled care in long-term care facilities either pay for it themselves or are on Medicaid. To ensure Medicaid reimbursement for these patients, you must document patient care once per day.

To secure payment for patients receiving intermediate care, you'll document medications and treatments daily. Document other types of care weekly, unless the patient's status changes and he requires a change in services. In this case, document the change and document his status more frequently. Also, perform a monthly reevaluation for these patients and an evaluation of expected outcomes for all Medicaid patients.

CMS

A branch of the Department of Health and Human Services, CMS regulates compliance with federal Medicare and Medicaid standards. CMS regulations are usually enforced at the state level.

To comply with CMS regulations, staff members at a long-term care facility must complete a lengthy form called the Minimum Data Set (MDS) for Resident Assessment and Care Screening, review the patient's status every 3 months, and perform a comprehensive reassessment annually.

OBRA

In 1987, Congress enacted OBRA, which imposed dozens of new requirements on long-term care facilities and home care agencies to protect the rights of patients receiving long-term care. OBRA requires that a comprehensive assessment be performed within 4 days of a patient's admission to a long-term care facility and then documented on the MDS form. The assessment and care screening process must be reviewed every 3 months and repeated annually — more often if the patient's condition changes.

In addition, a comprehensive nursing assessment and a formulated care plan must be completed. The comprehensive care plan must be completed within 7 days of the completion of the MDS. This date may vary depending on whether it's a Medicare Prospective Payment System (PPS) or an intermediate assessment.

JCAHO

JCAHO accredits long-term care facilities using standards developed in conjunction with health care experts. Standard performance is documented in assessments, progress notes, care plans, and discharge plans. The ORYX initiative, begun in 1997, is another part of the accreditation process. It focuses on outcomes and other performance measurement data. The purpose of the initiative is to support quality improvements, not just in long-term care but in all health care organizations.

Standard and required documents

Many forms are used in acute care and home care settings as well as in long-term care; others are used only in long-term care. Forms discussed in this chapter include:

- MDS
- Resident Assessment Protocol (RAP)
- Preadmission Screening and Annual Resident Review (PASARR)
- initial nursing assessment form
- nursing summaries
- ADL checklists and flow sheets
- care plans
- discharge and transfer forms.

In addition, many long-term care facilities have their own strict and comprehensive protocols. Typical protocols are those for bowel and bladder monitoring, physical and chemical restraints, safety, and infection control. Documentation requirements when using these protocols vary, so check your facility's policies.

MDS

Mandated by OBRA, the MDS is a federal regulatory form that must be filled out for every patient admitted to a long-term care facility. (See *Minimum Data Set form.*)

The MDS form proves compliance with performance improvement and reimbursement requirements, standardizes information, and helps health care team members and agencies communicate. Physicians, nurses, social workers, and other staff members complete and sign different sections of the form.

The requirements for completion of the MDS vary with the type of admission. For skilled care residents under PPS, Medicare requires completion at these times:

- 5-day assessment
- 14-day assessment
- 30-day assessment
- 60-day assessment

(Text continues on page 124.)

CHART QUICK

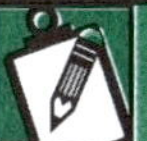

Minimum Data Set form

Patients in long-term care facilities that receive federal funds must have their health status evaluated at admission and a care plan devised. The patient's health status and care plan are revised every 7 days. The following is an excerpt of the Minimum Data Set form, which is used in its entirety for reevaluation.

Numeric Identifier________

MINIMUM DATA SET (MDS) — *VERSION 2.0*

FOR NURSING HOME RESIDENT ASSESSMENT AND CARE SCREENING

BASIC ASSESSMENT TRACKING FORM

SECTION AA. IDENTIFICATION INFORMATION

1.	RESIDENT NAME	Amy J Gaston a. (First) b. (Middle Initial) c. (Last) d. (Jr/Sr)
2.	GENDER	1. Male 2. Female — 2
3.	BIRTHDATE	12 – 30 – 1932 Month Day Year
4.	RACE/ETHNICITY	1. American Indian/Alaskan Native 2. Asian/Pacific Islander 3. Black, not of Hispanic origin 4. Hispanic 5. White, not of Hispanic origin — 5
5.	SOCIAL SECURITY AND MEDICARE NUMBERS [C in 1st box if non med. no.]	a. Social Security Number 041 – 24 – 0000 b. Medicare number (or comparable railroad insurance number)
6.	FACILITY PROVIDER NO.	a. State No. b. Federal No.
7.	MEDICAID NO. ["+" if pending, "N" if not a Medicaid recipient]	
8.	REASONS FOR ASSESSMENT	[Note—Other codes do not apply to this form] a. Primary reason for assessment — 1 1. Admission assessment (required by day 14) 2. Annual assessment 3. Significant change in status assessment 4. Significant correction of prior full assessment 5. Quarterly review assessment 10. Significant correction of prior quarterly assessment 0. NONE OF ABOVE b. *Codes for assessments required for Medicare PPS or the State* *1. Medicare 5 day assessment* *2. Medicare 30 day assessment* *3. Medicare 60 day assessment* *4. Medicare 90 day assessment* *5. Medicare readmission/return assessment* *6. Other state required assessment* *7. Medicare 14 day assessment* *8. Other Medicare required assessment*

9. Signatures of Persons who Completed a Portion of the Accompanying Assessment or Tracking Form

I certify that the accompanying information accurately reflects resident assessment or tracking information for this resident and that I collected or coordinated collection of this information on the dates specified. To the best of my knowledge, this information was collected in accordance with applicable Medicare and Medicaid requirements. I understand that this information is used as a basis for ensuring that residents receive appropriate and quality care, and as a basis for payment from federal funds. I further understand that payment of such federal funds and continued participation in the government-funded health care programs is conditioned on the accuracy and truthfulness of this information, and that I may be personally subject to or may subject my organization to substantial criminal, civil, and/or administrative penalties for submitting false information. I also certify that I am authorized to submit this information by this facility on its behalf.

	Signature and Title	Sections	Date
a.	Christine Saslo, RN, MSN		5/7/02
b.	Susan Rowe, MSN		
c.	James Shaw, RN, BSN		
d.			
e.			
f.			
g.			
h.			
i.			
j.			
k.			
l.			

GENERAL INSTRUCTIONS

Complete this information for submission with all full and quarterly assessments (Admission, Annual, Significant Change, State or Medicare required assessments, or Quarterly Reviews, etc.)

(continued)

Minimum Data Set form *(continued)*

Resident Amy J Gaston Numeric Identifier

MINIMUM DATA SET (MDS) *VERSION 2.0*

FOR NURSING HOME RESIDENT ASSESSMENT AND CARE SCREENING

BACKGROUND (FACE SHEET) INFORMATION AT ADMISSION

SECTION AB. DEMOGRAPHIC INFORMATION

1.	DATE OF ENTRY	*Date the stay began. Note — Does not include readmission if record was closed at time of temporary discharge to hospital, etc. In such cases, use prior admission date* 05-03-2002 (Month, Day, Year)	
2.	ADMITTED FROM (AT ENTRY)	1. Private home/apt. with no home health services 2. Private home/apt. with home health services 3. Board and care/assisted living/group home 4. Nursing home 5. Acute care hospital 6. Psychiatric hospital, MR/DD facility 7. Rehabilitation hospital 8. Other	1
3.	LIVED ALONE (PRIOR TO ENTRY)	0. No 1. Yes 2. In other facility	0
4.	ZIP CODE OF PRIOR PRIMARY RESIDENCE	19000	
5.	RESIDENTIAL HISTORY 5 YEARS PRIOR TO ENTRY	*(Check all settings resident lived in during 5 years prior to date of entry given in item AB1 above)* Prior stay at this nursing home a. Stay in other nursing home b. Other residential facility—board and care home, assisted living, group home c. MH/psychiatric setting d. MR/DD setting e. *NONE OF ABOVE* f.	
6.	LIFETIME OCCUPATION(S) [Put "/" between two occupations]	TEACHER	
7.	EDUCATION (*Highest Level Completed*)	1. No schooling 2. 8th grade/less 3. 9-11 grades 4. High school 5. Technical or trade school 6. Some college 7. Bachelor's degree 8. Graduate degree	8
8.	LANGUAGE	*(Code for correct response)* a. Primary Language 0. English 1. Spanish 2. French 3. Other b. If other, specify	0
9.	MENTAL HEALTH HISTORY	Does resident's RECORD indicate any history of mental retardation, mental illness, or developmental disability problem? 0. No 1. Yes	0
10.	CONDITIONS RELATED TO MR/DD STATUS	*(Check all conditions that are related to MR/DD status that were manifested before age 22, and are likely to continue indefinitely)* Not applicable—no MR/DD (Skip to AB11) a. √ MR/DD with organic condition Down's syndrome b. Autism c. Epilepsy d. Other organic condition related to MR/DD e. MR/DD with no organic condition f.	
11.	DATE BACKGROUND INFORMATION COMPLETED	05-07-2002 (Month, Day, Year)	

SECTION AC. CUSTOMARY ROUTINE

1. CUSTOMARY ROUTINE (*In year prior to DATE OF ENTRY to this nursing home, or year last in community if now being admitted from another nursing home*)

(Check all that apply. If all information UNKNOWN, check last box only.)

Item		Check
CYCLE OF DAILY EVENTS		
Stays up late at night (e.g., after 9 pm)	a.	
Naps regularly during day (at least 1 hour)	b.	√
Goes out 1+ days a week	c.	
Stays busy with hobbies, reading, or fixed daily routine	d.	√
Spends most of time alone or watching TV	e.	
Moves independently indoors (with appliances, if used)	f.	
Use of tobacco products at least daily	g.	
NONE OF ABOVE	h.	
EATING PATTERNS		
Distinct food preferences	i.	
Eats between meals all or most days	j.	√
Use of alcoholic beverage(s) at least weekly	k.	
NONE OF ABOVE	l.	
ADL PATTERNS		
In bedclothes much of day	m.	√
Wakens to toilet all or most nights	n.	
Has irregular bowel movement pattern	o.	
Showers for bathing	p.	
Bathing in PM	q.	√
NONE OF ABOVE	r.	
INVOLVEMENT PATTERNS		
Daily contact with relatives/close friends	s.	√
Usually attends church, temple, synagogue (etc.)	t.	
Finds strength in faith	u.	√
Daily animal companion/presence	v.	
Involved in group activities	w.	
NONE OF ABOVE	x.	
UNKNOWN—Resident/family unable to provide information	y.	

SECTION AD. FACE SHEET SIGNATURES

SIGNATURES OF PERSONS COMPLETING FACE SHEET:

Christine Saslo, RN, MSN

a. Signature of RN Assessment Coordinator Date

James Show, RN, BSN 5/7/02

I certify that the accompanying information accurately reflects resident assessment or tracking information for this resident and that I collected or coordinated collection of this information on the dates specified. To the best of my knowledge, this information was collected in accordance with applicable Medicare and Medicaid requirements. I understand that this information is used as a basis for ensuring that residents receive appropriate and quality care, and as a basis for payment from federal funds. I further understand that payment of such federal funds and continued participation in the government-funded health care programs is conditioned on the accuracy and truthfulness of this information, and that I may be personally subject to or may subject my organization to substantial criminal, civil, and/or administrative penalties for submitting false information. I also certify that I am authorized to submit this information by this facility on its behalf.

Signature and Title	Sections	Date
Susan Rowe, MSN		
b.		
c.		
d.		
e.		
f.		
g.		

☐ = When box blank, must enter number or letter [a.] = When letter in box, check if condition applies

MDS 2.0 September 2000

Minimum Data Set form *(continued)*

Resident Amy J Gaston Numeric Identifier

MINIMUM DATA SET (MDS) *VERSION 2.0*
FOR NURSING HOME RESIDENT ASSESSMENT AND CARE SCREENING
FULL ASSESSMENT FORM
(Status in last 7 days, unless other time frame indicated)

SECTION A. IDENTIFICATION AND BACKGROUND INFORMATION

1.	RESIDENT NAME	Amy J Gaston — a. (First) b. (Middle Initial) c. (Last) d. (Jr/Sr)	
2.	ROOM NUMBER	402	
3.	ASSESSMENT REFERENCE DATE	a. *Last day of MDS observation period* 05-07-2002 (Month Day Year) b. Original (0) or corrected copy of form (enter number of correction)	
4a.	DATE OF REENTRY	**Date of reentry from most recent temporary discharge to a hospital in last 90 days (or since last assessment or admission if less than 90 days)** ___-___-___ (Month Day Year)	
5.	MARITAL STATUS	1. Never married 2. Married 3. Widowed 4. Separated 5. Divorced	3
6.	MEDICAL RECORD NO.	MM000992268 1	
7.	CURRENT PAYMENT SOURCES FOR N.H. STAY	(*Billing Office to indicate; check all that apply in last 30 days*) Medicaid per diem a. Medicare per diem b. X Medicare ancillary part A c. Medicare ancillary part B d. CHAMPUS per diem e. VA per diem f. Self or family pays for full per diem g. X Medicaid resident liability or Medicare co-payment h. Private insurance per diem (including co-payment) i. Other per diem j.	
8.	REASONS FOR ASSESSMENT [*Note—If this is a discharge or reentry assessment, only a limited subset of MDS items need be completed*]	a. Primary reason for assessment 1. Admission assessment (required by day 14) 2. Annual assessment 3. Significant change in status assessment 4. Significant correction of prior full assessment 5. Quarterly review assessment 6. Discharged—return not anticipated 7. Discharged—return anticipated 8. Discharged prior to completing initial assessment 9. Reentry 10. Significant correction of prior quarterly assessment 0. *NONE OF ABOVE* **b. Codes for assessments required for Medicare PPS or the State** 1. *Medicare 5 day assessment* 2. *Medicare 30 day assessment* 3. *Medicare 60 day assessment* 4. *Medicare 90 day assessment* 5. *Medicare readmission/return assessment* 6. *Other state required assessment* 7. *Medicare 14 day assessment* 8. *Other Medicare required assessment*	a. 1
9.	RESPONSIBILITY/ LEGAL GUARDIAN	(*Check all that apply*) Legal guardian a. Other legal oversight b. Durable power of attorney/health care c. X Durable power attorney/financial d. Family member responsible e. Patient responsible for self f. *NONE OF ABOVE* g.	
10.	ADVANCED DIRECTIVES	(*For those items with supporting documentation in the medical record, check all that apply*) Living will a. X Do not resuscitate b. Do not hospitalize c. Organ donation d. Autopsy request e. Feeding restrictions f. Medication restrictions g. Other treatment restrictions h. *NONE OF ABOVE* i.	

SECTION B. COGNITIVE PATTERNS

1.	COMATOSE	(*Persistent vegetative state/no discernible consciousness*) 0. No 1. Yes **(If yes, skip to Section G)**	0
2.	MEMORY	(*Recall of what was learned or known*) a. Short-term memory OK—seems/appears to recall after 5 minutes 0. Memory OK 1. Memory problem	1
		b. Long-term memory OK—seems/appears to recall long past 0. Memory OK 1. Memory problem	1
3.	MEMORY/ RECALL ABILITY	(***Check all that resident was normally able to recall during last 7 days***) Current season a. Location of own room b. Staff names/faces c. That he/she is in a nursing home d. *NONE OF ABOVE* are recalled e. X	
4.	COGNITIVE SKILLS FOR DAILY DECISION-MAKING	(*Made decisions regarding tasks of daily life*) 0. *INDEPENDENT*—decisions consistent/reasonable 1. *MODIFIED INDEPENDENCE*—some difficulty in new situations only 2. *MODERATELY IMPAIRED*—decisions poor; cues/supervision required 3. *SEVERELY IMPAIRED*—never/rarely made decisions	2
5.	INDICATORS OF DELIRIUM—PERIODIC DISORDERED THINKING/ AWARENESS	(*Code for behavior in the last 7 days.*) [***Note: Accurate assessment requires conversations with staff and family who have direct knowledge of resident's behavior over this time***]. 0. Behavior not present 1. Behavior present, not of recent onset 2. Behavior present, over last 7 days appears different from resident's usual functioning (e.g., new onset or worsening)	
		a. EASILY DISTRACTED—(e.g., difficulty paying attention; gets sidetracked)	1
		b. PERIODS OF ALTERED PERCEPTION OR AWARENESS OF SURROUNDINGS—(e.g., moves lips or talks to someone not present; believes he/she is somewhere else; confuses night and day)	0
		c. EPISODES OF DISORGANIZED SPEECH—(e.g., speech is incoherent, nonsensical, irrelevant, or rambling from subject to subject; loses train of thought)	0
		d. PERIODS OF RESTLESSNESS—(e.g., fidgeting or picking at skin, clothing, napkins, etc; frequent position changes; repetitive physical movements or calling out)	0
		e. PERIODS OF LETHARGY—(e.g., sluggishness; staring into space; difficult to arouse; little body movement)	0
		f. MENTAL FUNCTION VARIES OVER THE COURSE OF THE DAY—(e.g., sometimes better, sometimes worse; behaviors sometimes present, sometimes not)	0
6.	CHANGE IN COGNITIVE STATUS	Resident's cognitive status, skills, or abilities have changed as compared to status of **90 days ago** (or since last assessment if less than 90 days) 0. No change 1. Improved 2. Deteriorated	0

SECTION C. COMMUNICATION/HEARING PATTERNS

1.	HEARING	(*With hearing appliance, if used*) 0. *HEARS ADEQUATELY*—normal talk, TV, phone 1. *MINIMAL DIFFICULTY* when not in quiet setting 2. *HEARS IN SPECIAL SITUATIONS ONLY*—speaker has to adjust tonal quality and speak distinctly 3. *HIGHLY IMPAIRED*/absence of useful hearing	1
2.	COMMUNICATION DEVICES/ TECHNIQUES	(*Check all that apply during last 7 days*) Hearing aid, present and used a. Hearing aid, present and not used regularly b. Other receptive comm. techniques used (e.g., lip reading) c. *NONE OF ABOVE* d. X	
3.	MODES OF EXPRESSION	(*Check all used by resident to make needs known*) Speech a. X Writing messages to express or clarify needs b. American sign language or Braille c. Signs/gestures/sounds d. Communication board e. Other f. *NONE OF ABOVE* g.	
4.	MAKING SELF UNDERSTOOD	(*Expressing information content—however able*) 0. *UNDERSTOOD* 1. *USUALLY UNDERSTOOD*—difficulty finding words or finishing thoughts 2. *SOMETIMES UNDERSTOOD*—ability is limited to making concrete requests 3. *RARELY/NEVER UNDERSTOOD*	1
5.	SPEECH CLARITY	(*Code for speech in the last 7 days*) 0. *CLEAR SPEECH*—distinct, intelligible words 1. *UNCLEAR SPEECH*—slurred, mumbled words 2. *NO SPEECH*—absence of spoken words	0
6.	ABILITY TO UNDERSTAND OTHERS	(*Understanding verbal information content—however able*) 0. *UNDERSTANDS* 1. *USUALLY UNDERSTANDS*—may miss some part/intent of message 2. *SOMETIMES UNDERSTANDS*—responds adequately to simple, direct communication 3. *RARELY/NEVER UNDERSTANDS*	2
7.	CHANGE IN COMMUNICATION/ HEARING	Resident's ability to express, understand, or hear information has changed as compared to status of **90 days ago** (or since last assessment if less than 90 days) 0. No change 1. Improved 2. Deteriorated	0

When box blank, must enter number or letter [a] = When letter in box, check if condition applies

MDS 2.0 September, 2000

(continued)

Minimum Data Set form *(continued)*

Resident *Amy J Gaston*   Numeric Identifier ____

SECTION D. VISION PATTERNS

1.	VISION	*(Ability to see in adequate light and with glasses if used)* 0. *ADEQUATE*—sees fine detail, including regular print in newspapers/books 1. *IMPAIRED*—sees large print, but not regular print in newspapers/books 2. *MODERATELY IMPAIRED*—limited vision; not able to see newspaper headlines, but can identify objects 3. *HIGHLY IMPAIRED*—object identification in question, but eyes appear to follow objects 4. *SEVERELY IMPAIRED*—no vision or sees only light, colors, or shapes; eyes do not appear to follow objects	0
2.	VISUAL LIMITATIONS/ DIFFICULTIES	Side vision problems—decreased peripheral vision (e.g., leaves food on one side of tray, difficulty traveling, bumps into people and objects, misjudges placement of chair when seating self)	a.
		Experiences any of following: sees halos or rings around lights; sees flashes of light; sees "curtains" over eyes	b.
		NONE OF ABOVE	c. X
3.	VISUAL APPLIANCES	Glasses; contact lenses; magnifying glass 0. No 1. Yes	1

SECTION E. MOOD AND BEHAVIOR PATTERNS

1.	INDICATORS OF DEPRESSION, ANXIETY, SAD MOOD	***(Code for indicators observed in last 30 days, irrespective of the assumed cause)*** 0. Indicator not exhibited in last 30 days 1. Indicator of this type exhibited up to five days a week 2. Indicator of this type exhibited daily or almost daily (6, 7 days a week)	

Indicator	Code	Indicator	Code
VERBAL EXPRESSIONS OF DISTRESS		h. Repetitive health complaints—e.g., persistently seeks medical attention, obsessive concern with body functions	0
a. Resident made negative statements—e.g., *"Nothing matters; Would rather be dead; What's the use; Regrets having lived so long; Let me die"*	0	i. Repetitive anxious complaints/concerns (non-health related) e.g., persistently seeks attention/ reassurance regarding schedules, meals, laundry, clothing, relationship issues	0
b. Repetitive questions—e.g., *"Where do I go; What do I do?"*	0	**SLEEP-CYCLE ISSUES**	
c. Repetitive verbalizations—e.g., calling out for help, (*"God help me"*)	0	j. Unpleasant mood in morning	0
d. Persistent anger with self or others—e.g., easily annoyed, anger at placement in nursing home; anger at care received	0	k. Insomnia/change in usual sleep pattern	0
		SAD, APATHETIC, ANXIOUS APPEARANCE	
e. Self deprecation—e.g., *"I am nothing; I am of no use to anyone"*	0	l. Sad, pained, worried facial expressions—e.g., furrowed brows	0
		m. Crying, tearfulness	0
f. Expressions of what appear to be unrealistic fears—e.g., fear of being abandoned, left alone, being with others	0	n. Repetitive physical movements—e.g., pacing, hand wringing, restlessness, fidgeting, picking	0
		LOSS OF INTEREST	
g. Recurrent statements that something terrible is about to happen—e.g., believes he or she is about to die, have a heart attack	0	o. Withdrawal from activities of interest—e.g., no interest in long standing activities or being with family/friends	0
		p. Reduced social interaction	0

2.	MOOD PERSISTENCE	**One or more indicators of depressed, sad or anxious mood were not easily altered by attempts to "cheer up", console, or reassure the resident over last 7 days** 0. No mood indicators 1. Indicators present, easily altered 2. Indicators present, not easily altered	0
3.	CHANGE IN MOOD	Resident's mood status has changed as compared to status of 90 days ago (or since last assessment if less than 90 days) 0. No change 1. Improved 2. Deteriorated	0
4.	BEHAVIORAL SYMPTOMS	***(A) Behavioral symptom frequency in last 7 days*** 0. Behavior not exhibited in last 7 days 1. Behavior of this type occurred 1 to 3 days in last 7 days 2. Behavior of this type occurred 4 to 6 days, but less than daily 3. Behavior of this type occurred daily ***(B) Behavioral symptom alterability in last 7 days*** 0. Behavior not present OR behavior was easily altered 1. Behavior was not easily altered	

Behavioral symptom	(A)	(B)
a. WANDERING (moved with no rational purpose, seemingly oblivious to needs or safety)	0	0
b. VERBALLY ABUSIVE BEHAVIORAL SYMPTOMS (others were threatened, screamed at, cursed at)	0	0
c. PHYSICALLY ABUSIVE BEHAVIORAL SYMPTOMS (others were hit, shoved, scratched, sexually abused)	0	0
d. SOCIALLY INAPPROPRIATE/DISRUPTIVE BEHAVIORAL SYMPTOMS (made disruptive sounds, noisiness, screaming, self-abusive acts, sexual behavior or disrobing in public, smeared/threw food/feces, hoarding, rummaged through others' belongings)	0	0
e. RESISTS CARE (resisted taking medications/ injections, ADL assistance, or eating)	0	0

5.	CHANGE IN BEHAVIORAL SYMPTOMS	Resident's behavior status has changed as compared to status of 90 days ago (or since last assessment if less than 90 days) 0. No change 1. Improved 2. Deteriorated	0

SECTION F. PSYCHOSOCIAL WELL-BEING

1.	SENSE OF INITIATIVE/ INVOLVEMENT	At ease interacting with others	a. X
		At ease doing planned or structured activities	b.
		At ease doing self-initiated activities	c.
		Establishes own goals	d.
		Pursues involvement in life of facility (e.g., makes/keeps friends; involved in group activities; responds positively to new activities; assists at religious services)	e.
		Accepts invitations into most group activities	f. X
		NONE OF ABOVE	g.
2.	UNSETTLED RELATIONSHIPS	Covert/open conflict with or repeated criticism of staff	a.
		Unhappy with roommate	b.
		Unhappy with residents other than roommate	c.
		Openly expresses conflict/anger with family/friends	d. X
		Absence of personal contact with family/friends	e.
		Recent loss of close family member/friend	f.
		Does not adjust easily to change in routines	g.
		NONE OF ABOVE	h.
3.	PAST ROLES	Strong identification with past roles and life status	a. X
		Expresses sadness/anger/empty feeling over lost roles/status	b.
		Resident perceives that daily routine (customary routine, activities) is very different from prior pattern in the community	c.
		NONE OF ABOVE	d.

SECTION G. PHYSICAL FUNCTIONING AND STRUCTURAL PROBLEMS

1. (A) ADL SELF-PERFORMANCE—***(Code for resident's PERFORMANCE OVER ALL SHIFTS during last 7 days—Not including setup)***

0. *INDEPENDENT*—No help or oversight —OR— Help/oversight provided only 1 or 2 times during last 7 days
1. *SUPERVISION*—Oversight, encouragement or cueing provided 3 or more times during last 7 days —OR— Supervision (3 or more times) plus physical assistance provided only 1 or 2 times during last 7 days
2. *LIMITED ASSISTANCE*—Resident highly involved in activity; received physical help in guided maneuvering of limbs or other nonweight bearing assistance 3 or more times —OR—More help provided only 1 or 2 times during last 7 days
3. *EXTENSIVE ASSISTANCE*—While resident performed part of activity, over last 7-day period, help of following type(s) provided 3 or more times:
   - Weight-bearing support
   - Full staff performance during part (but not all) of last 7 days
4. *TOTAL DEPENDENCE*—Full staff performance of activity during entire 7 days
8. *ACTIVITY DID NOT OCCUR* during entire 7 days

(B) ADL SUPPORT PROVIDED—***(Code for MOST SUPPORT PROVIDED OVER ALL SHIFTS during last 7 days; code regardless of resident's self-performance classification)***

0. No setup or physical help from staff
1. Setup help only
2. One person physical assist
3. Two+ persons physical assist
8. ADL activity itself did not occur during entire 7 days

			(A) SELF-PERF	(B) SUPPORT
a.	BED MOBILITY	How resident moves to and from lying position, turns side to side, and positions body while in bed	3	3
b.	TRANSFER	How resident moves between surfaces—to/from: bed, chair, wheelchair, standing position (EXCLUDE to/from bath/toilet)	4	3
c.	WALK IN ROOM	How resident walks between locations in his/her room	4	2
d.	WALK IN CORRIDOR	How resident walks in corridor on unit	4	3
e.	LOCOMOTION ON UNIT	How resident moves between locations in his/her room and adjacent corridor on same floor. If in wheelchair, self-sufficiency once in chair	4	2
f.	LOCOMOTION OFF UNIT	How resident moves to and returns from off unit locations (e.g., areas set aside for dining, activities, or treatments). **If facility has only one floor,** how resident moves to and from distant areas on the floor. If in wheelchair, self-sufficiency once in chair	4	2
g.	DRESSING	How resident puts on, fastens, and takes off all items of **street clothing**, including donning/removing prosthesis	4	3
h.	EATING	How resident eats and drinks (regardless of skill). Includes intake of nourishment by other means (e.g., tube feeding, total parenteral nutrition)	2	2
i.	TOILET USE	How resident uses the toilet room (or commode, bedpan, urinal); transfer on/off toilet, cleanses, changes pad, manages ostomy or catheter, adjusts clothes	4	3
j.	PERSONAL HYGIENE	How resident maintains personal hygiene, including combing hair, brushing teeth, shaving, applying makeup, washing/drying face, hands, and perineum (EXCLUDE baths and showers)	4	2

MDS 2.0 September, 2000

Minimum Data Set form (continued)

Resident: Amy J Gaston

Numeric Identifier

2.	BATHING	How resident takes full-body bath/shower, sponge bath, and transfers in/out of tub/shower (EXCLUDE washing of back and hair.) Code for most dependent in self-performance and support. (A) BATHING SELF-PERFORMANCE codes appear below 0. Independent—No help provided 1. Supervision—Oversight help only 2. Physical help limited to transfer only 3. Physical help in part of bathing activity 4. Total dependence 8. Activity itself did not occur during entire 7 days (Bathing support codes are as defined in Item 1, code B above)	(A) 4 (B) 3
3.	TEST FOR BALANCE (see training manual)	(Code for ability during test in the last 7 days) 0. Maintained position as required in test 1. Unsteady, but able to rebalance self without physical support 2. Partial physical support during test; or stands (sits) but does not follow directions for test 3. Not able to attempt test without physical help a. Balance while standing b. Balance while sitting—position, trunk control	a. 3 b. 2
4.	FUNCTIONAL LIMITATION IN RANGE OF MOTION (see training manual)	(Code for limitations during last 7 days that interfered with daily functions or placed resident at risk of injury) (A) RANGE OF MOTION: 0. No limitation; 1. Limitation on one side; 2. Limitation on both sides (B) VOLUNTARY MOVEMENT: 0. No loss; 1. Partial loss; 2. Full loss a. Neck b. Arm—Including shoulder or elbow c. Hand—Including wrist or fingers d. Leg—Including hip or knee e. Foot—Including ankle or toes f. Other limitation or loss	(A) (B) a. 1 1 b. 1 1 c. 1 1 d. 1 1 e. 1 1 f. 0 0
5.	MODES OF LOCOMOTION	(Check all that apply during last 7 days) Cane/walker/crutch a. Wheeled self b. Other person wheeled c. Wheelchair primary mode of locomotion d. X NONE OF ABOVE e.	
6.	MODES OF TRANSFER	(Check all that apply during last 7 days) Bedfast all or most of time a. X Bed rails used for bed mobility or transfer b. Lifted manually c. Lifted mechanically d. Transfer aid (e.g., slide board, trapeze, cane, walker, brace) e. NONE OF ABOVE f.	
7.	TASK SEGMENTATION	Some or all of ADL activities were broken into subtasks during last 7 days so that resident could perform them 0. No 1. Yes	0
8.	ADL FUNCTIONAL REHABILITATION POTENTIAL	Resident believes he/she is capable of increased independence in at least some ADLs a. Direct care staff believe resident is capable of increased independence in at least some ADLs b. Resident able to perform tasks/activity but is very slow c. Difference in ADL Self-Performance or ADL Support, comparing mornings to evenings d. NONE OF ABOVE e. 0	
9.	CHANGE IN ADL FUNCTION	Resident's ADL self-performance status has changed as compared to status of 90 days ago (or since last assessment if less than 90 days) 0. No change 1. Improved 2. Deteriorated	0

SECTION H. CONTINENCE IN LAST 14 DAYS

1.	CONTINENCE SELF-CONTROL CATEGORIES (Code for resident's PERFORMANCE OVER ALL SHIFTS)	0. CONTINENT—Complete control [includes use of indwelling urinary catheter or ostomy device that does not leak urine or stool] 1. USUALLY CONTINENT—BLADDER, incontinent episodes once a week or less; BOWEL, less than weekly 2. OCCASIONALLY INCONTINENT—BLADDER, 2 or more times a week but not daily; BOWEL, once a week 3. FREQUENTLY INCONTINENT—BLADDER, tended to be incontinent daily, but some control present (e.g., on day shift); BOWEL, 2-3 times a week 4. INCONTINENT—Had inadequate control BLADDER, multiple daily episodes; BOWEL, all (or almost all) of the time	
a.	BOWEL CONTINENCE	Control of bowel movement, with appliance or bowel continence programs, if employed	2
b.	BLADDER CONTINENCE	Control of urinary bladder function (if dribbles, volume insufficient to soak through underpants), with appliances (e.g., foley) or continence programs, if employed	2
2.	BOWEL ELIMINATION PATTERN	Bowel elimination pattern regular—at least one movement every three days a. X Constipation b. Diarrhea c. Fecal impaction d. NONE OF ABOVE e.	

3.	APPLIANCES AND PROGRAMS	Any scheduled toileting plan a. Bladder retraining program b. External (condom) catheter c. Indwelling catheter d. Intermittent catheter e. Did not use toilet room/commode/urinal f. Pads/briefs used g. X Enemas/irrigation h. Ostomy present i. NONE OF ABOVE j.	
4.	CHANGE IN URINARY CONTINENCE	Resident's urinary continence has changed as compared to status of 90 days ago (or since last assessment if less than 90 days) 0. No change 1. Improved 2. Deteriorated	0

SECTION I. DISEASE DIAGNOSES

Check only those diseases that have a relationship to current ADL status, cognitive status, mood and behavior status, medical treatments, nursing monitoring, or risk of death. (Do not list inactive diagnoses)

1.	DISEASES	(If none apply, CHECK the NONE OF ABOVE box) **ENDOCRINE/METABOLIC/NUTRITIONAL** Diabetes mellitus a. Hyperthyroidism b. Hypothyroidism c. X **HEART/CIRCULATION** Arteriosclerotic heart disease (ASHD) d. Cardiac dysrhythmias e. Congestive heart failure f. Deep vein thrombosis g. Hypertension h. Hypotension i. Peripheral vascular disease j. X Other cardiovascular disease k. **MUSCULOSKELETAL** Arthritis l. Hip fracture m. Missing limb (e.g., amputation) n. Osteoporosis o. Pathological bone fracture p. **NEUROLOGICAL** Alzheimer's disease q. Aphasia r. Cerebral palsy s. Cerebrovascular accident (stroke) t. Dementia other than Alzheimer's disease u. X Hemiplegia/Hemiparesis v. Multiple sclerosis w. Paraplegia x. Parkinson's disease y. Quadriplegia z. Seizure disorder aa. Transient ischemic attack (TIA) bb. Traumatic brain injury cc. **PSYCHIATRIC/MOOD** Anxiety disorder dd. Depression ee. Manic depression (bipolar disease) ff. Schizophrenia gg. **PULMONARY** Asthma hh. Emphysema/COPD ii. **SENSORY** Cataracts jj. Diabetic retinopathy kk. Glaucoma ll. Macular degeneration mm. **OTHER** Allergies nn. Anemia oo. Cancer pp. Renal failure qq. NONE OF ABOVE rr.
2.	INFECTIONS	(If none apply, CHECK the NONE OF ABOVE box) Antibiotic resistant infection (e.g., Methicillin resistant staph) a. Clostridium difficile (c. diff.) b. Conjunctivitis c. X HIV infection d. Pneumonia e. Respiratory infection f. Septicemia g. Sexually transmitted diseases h. Tuberculosis i. Urinary tract infection in last 30 days j. Viral hepatitis k. Wound infection l. NONE OF ABOVE m.
3.	OTHER CURRENT OR MORE DETAILED DIAGNOSES AND ICD-9 CODES	a. Hypertension 402.11 b. c. d. e.

- 90-day assessment
- readmission or return assessment.

For intermediate care residents, the MDS is completed at these times:

- admission assessment—required by day 14
- annual assessment
- significant change in status assessment
- quarterly review assessment—performed every 3 months.

RAP

Once an MDS form is completed, coded, computed, and processed, the patient's primary problems can be identified. These problems provide the basis for the patient's care plan. Another federally mandated form, the RAP summary, lists identified problem areas and documents the existence of a corresponding care plan. For example, if the patient has a stage 2 pressure ulcer documented in the MDS, the RAP summary indicates the need for a care plan to treat the pressure ulcer.

PASARR

For a patient to qualify for Medicare or Medicaid reimbursement, his mental status must also be documented. Federal regulations require that a long-term care facility performs a complete mental status assessment and documents it on a PASARR form. (See *PASARR identification form.*)

INITIAL NURSING ASSESSMENT

The required initial nursing assessment form is similar to the initial assessment form used in other settings. When documenting your initial assessment in a long-term care setting, be sure to place special emphasis on the patient's:

- activity level
- hearing and vision
- bowel and bladder control
- ability to communicate
- safety
- need for adaptive devices to assist dexterity and mobility
- family relationships
- transition from home or hospital to the long-term care facility.

NURSING SUMMARIES

Care and status updates must be completed regularly in long-term care facilities. Usually, you must complete a standard nursing care summary at least once every 2 to 4 weeks for patients with specific problems, such as pressure ulcers, who are receiving skilled care. A summary addressing the specific problems must be done weekly. For patients receiving intermediate care, a standard nursing care summary is usually required every 4 weeks.

The nursing summary describes:

- ability to perform ADLs
- nutrition and hydration
- safety measures, such as bed rails, restraints, and adaptive devices
- medications and other treatments
- problems adjusting to the long-term care facility.

In addition, you must complete a nursing assessment summary at least monthly to comply with Medicare and Medicaid standards.

ADL CHECKLISTS AND FLOW SHEETS

ADL checklists and flow sheets are forms that are usually completed by a nursing assistant or a restorative nurse on each shift; then you review and sign them. These forms tell the health care

(Text continues on page 128.)

CHART QUICK

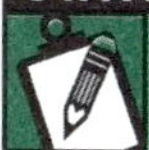

PASARR identification form

Before a patient covered by Medicare or Medicaid enters a long-term care facility, he must undergo an evaluation of mental status, using the Preadmission Screening and Annual Resident Review (PASARR) form, as shown here.

Section A: Identifying information for applicant/resident

LAST NAME: Perrone | FIRST NAME: Joseph | MI: R | MEDICAID RECIPIENT? N — Y = Yes N = No P = Pending

SEX: M — M = Male F = Female | DATE OF BIRTH: 08101933 | SOC SEC NO: 012345678

Section B: Reason for screening

ENTER CODE: 1

Preadmission Screening Codes	Annual Resident Review Codes	
1-Nursing facility applicant	3-Expired time limit for convalescent stay	6-Significant change in condition
2-PASSPORT waiver applicant	4-Expired time limit for emergency admission	7-No previous PASARR records
	5-Expired time limit for respite admission	8-ODMH use only
		9-Other

Section C: Dementia questions

YES ☑ NO ☐ (1) Does the individual have a documented PRIMARY diagnosis of dementia, Alzheimer's disease, or some other organic mental disorder as defined in *DSM-III-R*? If YES, the individual doesn't have indications of serious MI, go to Section E. If NO, go to the next question.

YES ☐ NO ☐ (2) Does the individual have a SECONDARY diagnosis of dementia, Alzheimer's disease, or some other organic mental disorder as defined in *DSM-III-R*? If YES, go to the next question. If NO, go to Section D.

YES ☐ NO ☐ (3) Does the individual have a PRIMARY diagnosis of one of the mental disorders listed in Question D(1) below? If YES, go to Section D. If NO, the individual doesn't have indications of serious MI, go to Section E.

Section D: Indications of serious mental illness

YES ☐ NO ☐ (1) Does the individual have a diagnosis of any of the mental disorders listed below? Check all that apply.

a. ☐ Schizophrenic disorder
b. ☐ Mood disorder
c. ☐ Delusional (paranoid) disorder
d. ☐ Panic or other severe anxiety disorder
e. ☐ Somatoform disorder
f. ☐ Personality disorder
g. ☐ Other psychotic disorder
h. ☐ Another mental disorder other than MR that may lead to a chronic disability
Describe: ____________

(continued)

PASARR identification form (continued)

Section D: Indications of serious mental illness *(continued)*

YES ☐ NO ☐ (2) Within the past 2 years, DUE TO THE MENTAL DISORDER, has the individual:

(a) Utilized intensive psychiatric services more than once? Indicate the number of times the individual utilized each service over the last 2 years (e.g., 0, 1, 2, 7 times).

a. ☐ Ongoing case management from an MH agency? ("1" if continuously receiving over the last 2 years.)
b. ☐ Emergency mental health services?
c. ☐ Number of admissions to inpatient hospital settings for psychiatric reasons?
d. ☐ Number of admissions to partial hospitalization treatment programs for psychiatric reasons?
e. ☐ Number of admissions to Residential Care Facilities (RCFs) providing MH services or operated by an MH agency?
f. ☐ TOTAL SCORE: If total score equals 2 or more, answer YES to Questions D(2). Regardless of score, answer Question D(2)(b)

OR

(b) Had a disruption to his/her usual living arrangement (e.g., arrest, eviction, inter- or intra-facility transfer, locked seclusion)?

☐ Yes ☐ No If YES, answer YES to Question D(2).

YES ☐ NO ☐ (3) Within the past 6 months, DUE TO THE MENTAL DISORDER, has the individual experienced one or more of the following functional limitations on a continuing or intermittent basis? Check all that apply.

a. ☐ Maintaining personal hygiene
b. ☐ Dressing self
c. ☐ Walking/getting around
d. ☐ Maintaining adequate diet
e. ☐ Preparing/obtaining own meals
f. ☐ Maintaining prescribed medication regimen
g. ☐ Performing household chores
h. ☐ Going shopping
i. ☐ Using available transportation
j. ☐ Managing available funds
k. ☐ Securing necessary support services
l. ☐ Verbalizing needs

YES ☐ NO ☐ (4) Within the past 2 years, has the individual received SSI or SSDI due to a mental impairment?

YES ☐ NO ☐ (5) Does the individual have indications of serious mental illness?
The individual has indications of serious mental illness if the individual received:

- Yes to AT LEAST 2 of Questions D(1), D(2), or D(3); OR
- Yes to Question D(4).

Section E: Indications of MR or related condition

YES ☐ NO ☑ (1) Does the individual have a diagnosis of MR (mild, moderate, severe, or profound as described in the *American Association of Mental Retardation's Manual on Classification in Mental Retardation,* 1989)?

YES ☐ NO ☑ (2) Does the individual have a severe, chronic disability that's attributable to a condition other than mental illness but is closely related to MR because this condition results in impairment of general intellectual functioning or adaptive behavior similar to that of a person with MR and requires treatment or services similar to those required for a person with MR? If YES, specify: ______________________________
If NO, go question E(6).

YES ☐ NO ☐ (3) Did the disability manifest symptoms before the individual's 22nd birthday?

YES ☐ NO ☐ (4) Is the disability likely to continue indefinitely?

PASARR identification form *(continued)*

Section E: Indications of MR or related condition *(continued)*

YES ☐ NO ☐ (5) Did the disability result in functional limitations, prior to age 22, in 3 or more of the following major life activities? Check all that apply.

a. ☐ Self-care
b. ☐ Mobility
c. ☐ Economic self-sufficiency
d. ☐ Understanding and use of language
e. ☐ Self-direction
f. ☐ Learning
g. ☐ Capacity for independent living

YES ☐ NO ☑ (6) Does the person currently receive services from the County Board of MR/DD?

YES ☐ NO ☑ (7) Does the person have indications of MR or a related condition?
The individual has indications of MR or a related condition if the individual received:

- Yes to Question E(1); OR
- Yes to all of the following in this Section; Questions 2, 3, 4, AND 5; OR
- Yes to Question E(6).

Section F: Submitter information/certification

In order to process the screen, the submitter must provide his/her name and address and sign below. If the individual has indications of serious MI (YES to D[5]) and/or MR or a related condition (YES to E[7)], submitters must also complete Section G. If the individual has indications of neither, submitters don't have to complete Section G. The NF may not admit or retain individuals with indications of serious MI and/or MR or a related condition without further review by ODMH and/or ODMR/DD (OAC Rules 5101:3-3-151 and 5101:3-3-152).

LAST NAME: Brown
FIRST NAME: Lisa

STREET ADDRESS: 456 Main Street

CITY: Springhouse
STATE: PA
ZIP: 19477

TELEPHONE NUMBER: (215) 999-9900

I understand that this screening information may be relied upon in the payment of claims that will be from Federal and State funds, and that any willful falsification, or concealment of a material fact, may be prosecuted under Federal and State laws. I certify that to the best of my knowledge, the foregoing information is true, accurate, and complete.

SIGNATURE: Lisa Brown
TITLE: RN
EMPLOYER: Sunnyside Care Facility
DATE: 06 (MONTH) 10 (DAY) 02 (YEAR)

Section G: Mailing addresses

Complete this section ONLY if the individual has indications of serious MI, MR, or a related condition.

(1) What address should be used for mailing results of the PASARR evaluation to the applicant/ resident?

IN CARE OF/

STREET ADDRESS

CITY
STATE
ZIP
first 4 letters of county of residence

(continued)

PASARR identification form *(continued)*

Section G: Mailing addresses *(continued)*

(2) Please provide the following information about the individual's attending physician:

LAST NAME | FIRST NAME

STREET ADDRESS

CITY | STATE | ZIP | TELEPHONE NUMBER ( )

(3) If the individual has a legal representative, please provide the following information about the representative:

LAST NAME | FIRST NAME

STREET ADDRESS

CITY | STATE | ZIP | TELEPHONE NUMBER ( )

(4) If the individual is an applicant to or resident of an NF, please provide the name and address of the NF:

NAME OF NF

STREET ADDRESS

CITY | STATE | ZIP | first 4 letters of county

(5) If the individual is being discharged from a hospital, and the submitter isn't employed by the discharging hospital, please provide the name of a contact person and the name and address of the discharging hospital:

LAST NAME | FIRST NAME

STREET ADDRESS

CITY | STATE | ZIP | TELEPHONE NUMBER ( )

team members about the patient's abilities, degree of independence, and special needs so they can determine the type of assistance he requires.

The following tools are examples of checklists and flow sheets that can be used to assess ADLs:

- Katz index
- Lawton scale
- Barthel index and scale.

Katz index

The Katz index ranks the patient's ability in six areas:

- bathing
- dressing
- toileting
- moving from wheelchair to bed and returning
- continence
- feeding.

It describes the patient's functional level at a specific time and rates his

CHART QUICK

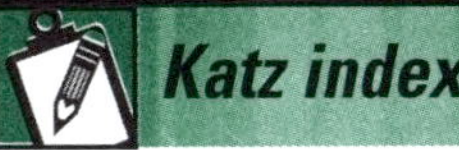

Katz index

The Katz index, shown below, is used to assess six basic activities of daily living.

EVALUATION FORM

Name *Henry Dancer* Date *06/18/02*

For each area of functioning listed below, check the description that applies. (The word "assistance" means supervision, direction, or personal assistance.)

Bathing: Sponge bath, tub bath, or shower.

☐ Receives no assistance; gets into and out of tub, if tub is usual means of bathing.	☑ Receives assistance in bathing only one part of the body, such as the back or leg.	○ Receives assistance in bathing more than one part of the body, or can't bathe.

Dressing: Gets outer garments and underwear from closets and drawers and uses fasteners, including suspenders, if worn.

☐ Gets clothes and gets completely dressed without assistance.	☐ Gets clothes and gets dressed without assistance except for tying shoes.	✓ Receives assistance in getting clothes or in getting dressed, or stays partly or completely undressed.

Toileting: Goes to the room termed "toilet" for bowel movement and urination, cleans self afterward, and arranges clothes.

☐ Goes to toilet room, cleans self, and arranges clothes without assistance. May use object for support, such as cane, walker, or wheelchair, and may manage night bedpan or commode, emptying it in the morning.	✓ Receives assistance in going to toilet room or in cleaning self or arranging clothes after elimination or in use of night bedpan or commode.	○ Doesn't go to toilet room for the elimination process.

Transfer

☐ Moves into and out of bed and chair without assistance. May use object, such as cane or walker for support.	✓ Moves into or out of bed or chair with assistance.	○ Doesn't get out of bed.

Continence

☑ Controls urination and bowel movement completely by self.	○ Has occasional accidents.	○ Supervision helps keep control of urination or bowel movement, or catheter is used, or is incontinent.

Feeding

☐ Feeds self without assistance.	☑ Feeds self except for assistance in cutting meat or buttering bread.	○ Receives assistance in feeding or is fed partly or completely through tubes or by I.V. fluids.

(continued)

Katz index *(continued)*

Evaluator: Germaine Fried, RN

Index

☐ Indicates independence
○ Indicates dependence

A: Independent in all six functions.
B: Independent in all but one of these functions.
C: Independent in all but bathing and one additional function.
D: Independent in all but bathing, dressing, and one additional function.
E: Independent in all but bathing, dressing, toileting, and one additional function.
F: Independent in all but bathing, dressing, toileting, transferring, and one additional function.
G: Dependent in all six functions.
Other: Dependent in at least two functions but not classifiable as C, D, E, or F.

performance of each function on three levels: performing without help, needing some help, or having complete disability. (See *Katz index,* pages 129 and 130.)

Lawton scale

The Lawton scale evaluates the patient's ability to perform complex personal care activities necessary for independent living. Activities include:

- using the telephone
- cooking
- shopping
- doing laundry
- managing finances
- taking medications
- preparing meals.

Activities are rated on a three-point scale, ranging from without help (3), to needing some help (2), to complete disability (1). (See *Lawton scale.*)

Barthel index and scale

The Barthel index and scale is used to evaluate:

- feeding
- moving from wheelchair to bed and returning
- performing personal hygiene
- getting on and off the toilet
- bathing
- walking on a level surface or propelling a wheelchair
- going up and down stairs
- dressing and undressing
- maintaining bowel continence
- controlling the bladder.

Each item is scored according to the amount of assistance needed. Over time, results reveal improvement or decline. Another scale, the Barthel Self-Care Rating Scale, evaluates function in greater detail. (See *Barthel index,* pages 132 and 133.)

CARE PLANS

Standards for care plans are developed by individual long-term care facilities. When a patient is admitted to a facility, an interim care plan is used until an interdisciplinary care conference regarding the patient takes place. The interim care plan should be in place within 24

CHART QUICK

Lawton scale

The Lawton scale, shown below, provides information about a patient's ability to perform more sophisticated tasks than basic activities of daily living.

Name *John Shapiro* Rated by *James Mott, RN* Date *April 8, 2002*

1. **Can you use the telephone?**
   without help .... (3)
   with some help 2
   completely unable 1

2. **Can you get to places beyond walking distance?**
   without help 3
   with some help .... (2)
   not without special arrangements 1

3. **Can you go shopping for groceries?**
   without help 3
   with some help .... (2)
   completely unable 1

4. **Can you prepare your own meals?**
   without help .... (3)
   with some help 2
   completely unable 1

5. **Can you do your own housework?**
   without help .... (3)
   with some help 2
   completely unable 1

6. **Can you do your own handyman work?**
   without help 3
   with some help .... (2)
   completely unable 1

7. **Can you do your own laundry?**
   without help .... (3)
   with some help 2
   completely unable 1

8a. **Do you take or use any medications?**
   Yes (If yes, answer question 8b.) .... (1)
   No (If no, answer question 8c.) 2

8b. **Do you take your own medicine?**
   without help (in the right doses at the right times) .... (3)
   with some help (if someone prepares it for you or reminds you to take it) 2
   completely unable 1

8c. **If you had to take medicine, could you do it?**
   without help (in the right doses at the right time) 3
   with some help (if someone prepared it for you or reminded you to take it) 2
   completely unable 1

9. **Can you manage your own money?**
   without help .... (3)
   with some help 2
   completely unable 1

The first answer in each question, except for 8a, indicates independence; the second indicates capability with assistance; and the third, dependence. In this version the maximum score is 29, although scores have meaning only for a particular patient such as when declining scores over time reveal deterioration.

Adapted with permission from Lawton, M.P., and Brody, E.M., "Assessment of Older People: Self-Maintaining and Instrumental Activities of Daily Living," *The Gerontologist* 9(3):179-86, Autumn 1969.

hours of admission. After this, a full care plan is developed for the patient. This interdisciplinary care plan should be completed within 7 days of the completion of the MDS. A documented review of the plan must be completed every 3 months or when the patient's status changes.

In long-term care settings, care plans usually evolve from an interdiscipli-

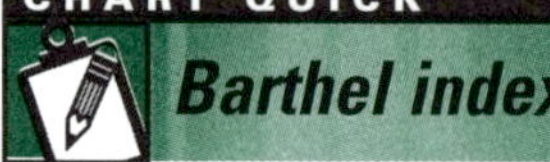

CHART QUICK

Barthel index

The Barthel index shown below is used to assess the patient's ability to perform 10 activities of daily living, document findings for other health care team members, and reveal improvement or decline.

Date *06/26/02*

Patient's name *Jack Boyd*

Evaluator *Kate Roth, RN*

Action	With help	Independent
Feeding (if food needs to be cut up = help)	5	**10**
Moving from wheelchair to bed and return (includes sitting up in bed)	5 to **10**	15
Personal toilet (wash face, comb hair, shave, clean teeth)	0	**5**
Getting on and off toilet (handling clothes, wipe, flush)	**5**	10
Bathing self	0	**5**
Walking on level surface (or, if unable to walk, propelling wheelchair)	0	**5** or 15
Ascending and descending stairs	**5**	10
Dressing (includes tying shoes, fastening fasteners)	**5**	10
Controlling bowels	5	**10**
Controlling bladder	**5**	10

Definition and Discussion of Scoring

A person scoring 100 is continent, feeds himself, dresses himself, gets up out of bed and chairs, bathes himself, walks at least a block, and can ascend and descend stairs. This doesn't mean that he's able to live alone; he may not be able to cook, keep house, or meet the public, but he's able to get along without attendant care.

Feeding

10 = Independent. The person can feed himself a meal from a tray or table when someone puts the food within his reach. He must be able to put on an assistive device if needed, cut up the food, use salt and pepper, spread butter, and so forth. Also, he must accomplish these tasks in a reasonable time.

5 = The person needs some help with cutting up food and other tasks, as listed above.

Moving from wheelchair to bed and return

15 = The person operates independently in all phases of this activity. He can safely approach the bed in his wheelchair, lock brakes, lift footrests, move safely from bed, lie down, come to a sitting position on the side of the bed, change the position of the wheelchair, if necessary, to transfer back into it safely, and return to the wheelchair.

10 = Either the person needs some minimal help in some step of this activity, or needs to be reminded or supervised for safety in one or more parts of this activity.

5 = The person can come to a sitting position without the help of a second person but needs to be lifted out of bed, or needs a great deal of help with transfers.

Handling personal toilet

5 = The person can wash hands and face, comb hair, clean teeth, and shave. He may use any kind of razor but he must be able to get it from the drawer or cabinet and plug it in or put in a blade without help. A female must put on her own makeup, if any, but need not braid or style her hair.

Barthel index *(continued)*

Getting on and off toilet

10 = The person is able to get on and off the toilet, unfasten and refasten clothes, prevent soiling of clothes, and use toilet paper without help. He may use a wall bar or other stable object for support, if needed. If he needs to use a bed pan instead of toilet, he must be able to place it on a chair, use it competently, and empty and clean it.

5 = The person needs help to overcome imbalance, handle clothes, or use toilet paper.

Bathing self

5 = The person may use a bath tub or shower or give himself a complete sponge bath. Regardless of method, he must be able to complete all the steps involved without another person's presence.

Walking on a level surface

15 = The person can walk at least 50 yards without help or supervision. He may wear braces or prostheses and use crutches, canes, or a walkerette, but not a rolling walker. He must be able to lock and unlock braces, if used, get the necessary mechanical aids into position for use, stand up and sit down, and dispose of the aids when he sits. (Putting on, fastening, and taking off braces is scored under Dressing).

5 = If the person can't ambulate but can propel a wheelchair independently, he must be able to go around corners, turn around, maneuver the chair to table, bed, toilet, and other locations. He must be able to push a chair at least 150′ (45.5 m). Don't score this item if the person receives a score for walking.

0 = Unable to walk.

Ascending and descending stairs

10 = The person can go up and down a flight of stairs safely without help or supervision. He may and should use handrails, canes, or crutches when needed, and he must be able to carry canes or crutches as he ascends or descends.

5 = The person needs help with or supervision of any one of the above items.

Dressing and undressing

10 = The person can put on, fasten, and remove all clothing (including any prescribed corset or braces) and tie shoe laces (unless he requires adaptations for this). Such special clothing as suspenders, loafers, and dresses that open down the front may be used when necessary.

5 = The person needs help in putting on, fastening, or removing any clothing. He must do at least half the work himself and must accomplish the task in a reasonable time. Women need not be scored on use of a brassiere or girdle unless these are prescribed garments.

Controlling bowels

10 = The person can control his bowels without accidents. He can use a suppository or take an enema when necessary (as in spinal cord injury patients who have had bowel training).

5 = The person needs help in using a suppository or taking an enema or has occasional accidents.

Controlling bladder

10 = The person can control his bladder day and night. Spinal cord injury patients who wear an external device and leg bag must put them on independently, clean and empty the bag, and stay dry, day and night.

5 = The person has occasional accidents, can't wait for the bed pan or get to the toilet in time, or needs help with an external device.

The total score is less significant or meaningful than the individual items, because these indicate where the deficiencies lie.

Any applicant to a long-term care facility who scores 100 should be evaluated carefully before admission to see whether admission is indicated. Discharged patients with scores of 100 shouldn't require further physical therapy but may benefit from a home visit to see whether any environmental adjustments are needed.

Adapted with permission from Mahoney, F.I., and Barthel, D.W. "Functional Evaluation: The Barthel Index," *Maryland State Medical Journal* 14:62, 1965.

nary approach to care, with contributions by the patient, his family members, and other health care providers.

As always, base your care plan on the patient's health problems, nursing diagnoses, and expected treatment outcomes. Include measurable patient outcomes with reasonable time frames and specific interventions to achieve them.

DISCHARGE AND TRANSFER FORMS

When the facility discharges a patient to home or a hospital, you must document the reason for discharge, the patient's destination, his mode of transportation, and the person or staff member accompanying him, if appropriate.

Other important data to include in this document are a list of prescribed medications, skin assessment findings, overall condition, disposition of personal belongings, and teaching topics that you covered (such as diet, medications, skin care, and other areas).

Guidelines drawn up by JCAHO emphasize the need to assess and summarize the patient's condition at transfer time. (See *Transfer and personal belongings form.*)

Documentation guidelines

In long-term care facilities, consider the following points when updating your records:

- When writing nursing summaries, address specific patient problems noted in the care plan.
- When writing progress notes, confirm that the patient's progress is being evaluated and reevaluated in relation to the goals or outcomes in the care plan. If goals aren't met, address this. Also, describe and document additional actions.
- Record transfers and discharges according to facility protocol.
- Document changes in the patient's condition and report them to the physician and the patient's family within 24 hours.
- Document follow-up interventions or other measures taken in response to a change in the patient's condition.
- Keep a record of visits from family or friends and of phone calls about the patient. State or federal regulators may fine your facility if these aren't documented.
- If an incident occurs, such as a fall or a treatment error, fill out an incident report and write follow-up notes for at least 48 hours after the incident (or follow your facility's policy).
- During the patient's first week of residence, keep detailed records on each shift.
- Flag a new patient by putting a red dot on the chart, bed, or door, or by using a similar system so that all staff members are aware of the new resident and become familiar with him. (Remember, however, to be sensitive to each patient's need for confidentiality and dignity.)
- Keep reimbursement in mind when documenting. For a facility to qualify for payment, its records must clearly reflect the level of care given to the patient.
- Make sure your records accurately reflect skilled services the patient receives.

CHART QUICK

Transfer and personal belongings form

Patients in long-term care facilities may be admitted to the hospital, discharged to home, or transferred to another facility. The form below is used during this process.

1. Patient's last name: *Clark* | First name: *Robert* | MI: *T*
2. Sex: *Male*
3. Social security number: *144-44-4444*

4. Patient's address (Street, City, State, Zip code): *1 Wise Street Springhouse, PA 19477*
5. Date of birth: *2-8-28*
6. Religion: *unknown*

7. Date of this transfer: *04/28/02*
8. Facility name and address transferring to: *Seniors Care Facility, 22 Elderly Way Philadelphia, PA*
9. Physician in charge at time of transfer: *Dr. Nicholas*
Will this physician care for patient after admission to new facility?
☐ Yes ☑ No

10. Dates of stay at facility transferring from
Admission: *04/22/02* Discharge: *04/28/02*

11. Payment source for charges to patient
A. ☑ Self or family
B. ☐ Private insurance
C. ☐ Blue Cross Blue Shield
D. ☐ Employer or union
E. ☐ Public agency (Give name)
F. ☐ Other (Explain)

12A. Name and address of facility transferring from: *Community Hospital, 3000 Medical Way Philadelphia, PA*
12B. Names and addresses of all hospitals and extended care facilities from which patient was discharged in past 60 days.

13. Clinic appointment Date Time Clinic appointment card attached
14. Date of last physical examination: *04/27/02*

15. Relative or guardian: Name: *Katherine Clark* Address: *1 Wise Street Springhouse, PA 19477* Phone number: *215-999-9000*

16. Diagnoses at time of transfer
(a) Primary *Ⓡ CVA*
(b) Secondary *IDDM*
Employment related: ☐ Yes ☑ No

Vitals at time of transfer
T *99* P *68* R *26* B/P *140/82*

Advance directives ☐ Yes ☑ No ☐ Copy attached
Code status *Full code*

Check all that apply

Disabilities
☐ Amputation
☑ Paralysis *Ⓛ side*
☐ Contracture
☐ Pressure ulcer

Impairments
☐ Mental
☑ Speech
☐ Hearing
☑ Vision
☐ Sensation

Incontinence
☑ Bladder
☑ Bowel
☑ Saliva

Activity tolerance limitations
☑ None
☐ Moderate
☐ Severe

Patient knows diagnosis
☑ Yes
☐ No

Potential for rehabilitation
☐ Good
☑ Fair
☐ Poor

Important medical information (State allergies if any)
PCN

Diet, drugs, and other therapy at time of discharge
-Mechanical soft diet (2,000 cal)
-Megace 4 tabs Q6h
-Lasix 40 mg P.O. b.i.d.
-Aspirin 81mg P.O. q.d.
-Humulin 70/30 20 units q a.m. & h.s.
-Sliding scale coverage: BS <40 >400
-Call Dr. Nicholas,
BS 200-250:2U / 301-350:4U
251-300:3U / 351-400:5U } Humulin R

(Physician, please sign below)
Henry C. Nicholas, MD

(continued)

Transfer and personal belongings form (continued)

Suggestions for active care

Bed
Position in good body alignment and change position every _2_ hrs.
Avoid _flat supine_ position. Prone position _2_ time/day as tolerated.

Sitting
_4_ hr _3_ times/day

Weight bearing
☐ Full
☑ Partial
☐ None
on ___ leg

Exercises
Range of motion _3_ times/day.
to _(L) extremities_ by
☐ patient ☐ nurse ☐ family
Stand _3_ min. _2_ times/day.

Locomotion
Walk _unable_ times/day.

Social activities
Encourage (☑ Group ☐ Individual) activities (☑ within ☐ outside) home.

Transportation
☑ Ambulance ☐ Car
☐ Car for handicapped ☐ Bus

Signature of physician or nurse _John Brown, RN_ Date _04/28/02_

Any articles of clothing or other belongings left at the hospital will be held for 30 days after discharge. Items remaining after this period will be disposed of by the hospital.

	Describe	✓	Comments
Date:	04/28/02		
Initials:			
Valuables	**Describe**		
Wallet:		✓	1 brown leather wallet
Money (Amount):	$25.00	✓	1 $20.00 bill, 5 $1.00 bills
Watch:			
Jewelry:			
Glasses/Contacts:	glasses	✓	wire rim – gold
Hearing Aids:			
Dentures:		✓	
Partial			
Complete		✓	container labeled
Keys:			
Article	**Describe**		
Ambulatory aids:			
Cane, walker, etc.			
Bedclothes:		✓	1 pair plaid pajamas
Belt:			
Dress:			
Outer wear:			
Pants:			
Pocketbook:			
Shirt:			
Shoes:			
Sweater:			
Undergarments:			
Other:			

All belongings were sent home with patient's family: Yes (No)

Patient' signature _Bob Clark_

Witnessed by hospital personnel _Mary Jones, RN_

- Always record a physician's verbal and telephone orders and have the physician countersign within 48 hours.
- Document visits by the physician to the patient. Generally accepted standards require one visit after admission, another after the first 30 days, and at

least one every 60 days thereafter. However, the resident's condition ultimately guides the frequency of physician visits.

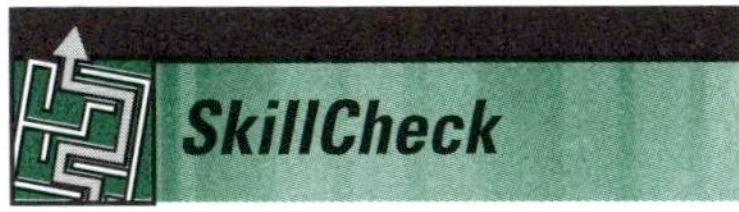

1. Which long-term care form is used to identify the patient's primary problems?
  a. MDS
  b. RAP
  c. PASARR
  d. Nursing summary

Answer: b. The RAP form lists the patient's identified problem areas and documents the existence of a corresponding care plan.

2. Which ADL checklist rates the patient's ability to perform basic tasks?
  a. Katz index
  b. Lawton scale
  c. Barthel index
  d. Initial nursing assessment form

Answer: a. The Katz index is used to assess the patient's ability to perform six basic ADLs and rates his performance of each function on three levels.

3. Which government regulation mandates that the MDS form be completed in long-term care facilities?
  a. Medicare
  b. Medicaid
  c. OBRA
  d. CMS

Answer: c. OBRA mandates that this federal regulatory form must be filled out for every patient admitted to a long-term care facility.

4. What are the two levels of care offered in long-term care facilities?
  a. Acute care and primary care
  b. Pediatric care and geriatric care
  c. Skilled care and intermediate care
  d. Home care and hospice care

Answer: c. Skilled care and intermediate care are the main levels of care offered in long-term care. The patient's needs determine which level of care he will require.

5. Which long-term care form is used to screen a patient's mental status?
  a. MDS
  b. RAP
  c. PASARR
  d. Lawton scale

Answer: c. Federal regulations require the PASARR form in long-term care to document complete mental status assessments for each patient.

6 Documenting in home care

The purpose of home care nursing is to restore, maintain, or promote health and function for a patient and his family at home. A home care agency plans, coordinates, and supplies care based on the needs of the patient and his family and the resources available to them. Home care is one component of comprehensive health care.

Recent trends have contributed to the growth of the home care industry, including:

- development of a prospective payment system (PPS) for home care agencies
- use of the Outcome and Assessment Information Set (OASIS), a tool used to help assess the patient's condition
- increased number of patients of advanced age
- increased availability of sophisticated home care equipment
- use of electronic claim processing and surveillance of the Centers for Medicare & Medicaid Services (CMS) and fiscal intermediaries.

The Balanced Budget Act of 1997 required the development of a PPS for Medicare home care services and the implementation of this system in October 2000. Under this system, Medicare will pay home care agencies a predetermined base payment. The payment will be adjusted for the health care needs and conditions of the patient.

Managed care organizations have identified sophisticated methods of performing utilization review, causing a decrease in the average length of stay. Therefore, a patient today is typically sicker when he's discharged to home.

Because support services in the home and community cost less than institutional care, government and private insurance payers are expanding their coverage of home care. In the future, the home care industry may become the primary supplier of health care in the United States.

Traditionally, homebound Medicare recipients have constituted the major portion of the home care caseload. Agencies have expanded services to new populations, representing all age-groups and a variety of medical conditions. This has led to the emergence of home care subspecialties, such as home infusion agencies and high-tech cancer-related home care, including stem cell transplants. These agencies may be offshoots of parent organizations or standalone agencies. (See *Hospice care services.*)

OASIS required

Although Medicare has tied reimbursement to the OASIS assessment, all patients older than age 18, excluding

Hospice care services

Many home care agencies provide hospice care services. Hospice programs provide palliative care to the terminally ill in the home and hospital.

Medicare coverage

Since 1983, a patient who has met specific admission criteria can qualify for the hospice Medicare benefit instead of the traditional Medicare benefit, allowing greater freedom to choose the hospice alternative for terminal care. The patient receives noncurative medical and support service not otherwise covered by Medicare.

Medicare coverage for hospice care is available if:

- The patient is eligible for Medicare Part A, which covers skilled nursing home and hospital care. People eligible for Medicare are those age 65 or older, long-term disabled patients, and people with end-stage renal disease.
- The patient's physician and the hospice medical director certify that the patient is terminally ill with a life expectancy of 6 months or less.
- The patient receives care from a Medicare-approved hospice program.

A Medicare-approved hospice will usually provide care in the patient's home. The hospice team and the patient's physician establish a care plan for medical and support services for the management of a terminal illness.

A patient without coverage for hospice benefits may be eligible for free or reduced-cost care through local programs or foundations. Alternatively, a patient may pay privately for hospice services.

Understanding and acceptance of treatment

With hospice care, the patient and primary caregiver must complete documentation indicating their understanding of hospice care. The patient and caregiver must sign an informed consent form that outlines everyone's responsibilities. The patient and primary caregiver must also sign a form indicating understanding and acceptance of the role of the primary caregiver.

women receiving maternal-child services, must have an OASIS evaluation. OASIS regulations require that nurses complete an assessment and agencies transmit the assessment and other data within strict time frames.

Patient assessment must be completed:

- within 5 days of the initiation of care and at 60 days and 120 days (if needed)
- when the patient is transferred to another agency
- when the patient is discharged from home care
- when there's a significant change in the patient's condition.

Before receiving care from a home care agency, a patient with private insurance must obtain authorization from his insurance provider. In many cases, insurance limitations restrict treatment options.

In this cost-conscious environment, nurses take on an especially important role in helping a patient get coverage by educating him about local, state, and federal benefit programs. When you help a patient identify a program for which he qualifies, such as veterans' benefits or Meals On Wheels, you help him get the services he needs while ensuring that your agency receives proper reimbursement.

Legal risks and responsibilities

Home care agencies are licensed and regulated by state governments and accredited by private agencies such as the Community Health Accreditation Program (CHAP), which is administered through the National League for Nursing (NLN) and the Joint Commission on Accreditation of Healthcare Organizations (JCAHO). In many cases, obtaining state licensure hinges on having accreditation. Home care agencies must also adhere to Medicare and Medicaid regulations administered by CMS and its agencies and carriers.

Home care agencies are evaluated for such factors as accurate and complete documentation and adherence to standards, particularly establishing eligibility for services and quality of care. If standards aren't met, a home care agency may fail to earn licensure or accreditation, may have its current license and accreditation revoked, or may have reimbursement privileges withheld or revoked.

RISKS OF POOR DOCUMENTATION

Home care agencies must maintain complete and legally sound documentation. For reimbursable services, nurses must document each instance that the specified service is provided. Nurses must also document the services the agency refuses to provide. Inadequate or incomplete documentation can have serious consequences.

Evaluating admissions

Since the inception of PPS for home care agencies, agencies have had to carefully evaluate admissions. Because of this evaluation process, not all patients who are referred for home care qualify. If a patient has no caregiver or has a complex chronic medical condition, the cost of his care may quickly exceed the allotted reimbursement. Therefore, home care agencies are unable to admit these patients.

A complete admission assessment and detailed documentation of this assessment are crucial in determining the appropriateness of each patient referred for admission.

Liability

After a nurse or home care agency is named in a lawsuit, it's too late to correct inaccurate documentation. For example, a nurse fails to record the patient's apical pulse and rhythm before administering digoxin. Later, the family sues the home care agency, alleging the staff caused the patient to go into complete heart block by failing to recognize signs of digoxin toxicity. Without a documented record, the agency can't prove that the patient wasn't experiencing excessive slowing of the pulse, a classic sign of digoxin toxicity.

Financial losses

Inadequate or incomplete documentation may result in refusal by third-party

Qualification criteria

Careful screening, which is done at the initial evaluation, is critical when determining what clinical services a patient needs. When evaluating a new patient for service, look for the following criteria.

Clinical criteria
- Skilled care needed
- Appropriately prescribed therapy that can be done in the home
- Caregiver available to assist patient

Technical criteria (patient or caregiver)
- Intact senses
- Capability of learning and following procedures
- Capability of recognizing complications and initiating emergency medical procedures

Environmental criteria
- Access to a telephone
- Access to electricity
- Access to water
- Clean living environment

Financial criteria
- Verification of insurance coverage
- Full knowledge of copayment or out-of-pocket expenses
- Agreement to comply with conditions of participation

payers or fiscal intermediaries to cover services. Insurance companies that negotiate preferred provider contracts may refuse to do business with home care agencies that provide incomplete documentation.

DOCUMENTATION GUIDELINES

Documentation of care and discharge planning begins when you evaluate a new patient for service. (See *Qualification criteria.*) You may use a referral form to document the patient's needs. (See *Referral form,* page 142.) Patients and caregivers also fill out several forms during the initial home visit. These required forms include patient rights and responsibilities; advance directives, including a do-not-resuscitate option; consent for services; medical information authorization and release; assignment of benefits; equipment acceptance; and a patient teaching checklist. If the patient requires an I.V. infusion, the forms also include consent for vascular access and an infusion treatment service agreement.

When you start caring for a patient, always document activities completed during your nursing visit, such as assessments and interventions, the patient's response to treatment, and whether he experienced complications. Also, record your communications with other members of the health care team and the date of the next visit. Use your agency's flow sheets.

The information you provide is used by third-party payers during utilization review to evaluate each claim in accordance with criteria for coverage. It may also be used by the government and oversight agencies to determine the validity of services.

Home care documentation should cover:

- OASIS

CHART QUICK

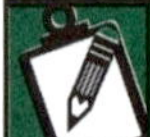

Referral form

Also called an intake form, this form is used to document the patient's needs when you begin your evaluation of a new patient. The sample below is a portion of such a form.

Date of referral: *6/17/02* Branch: *North* Chart #: *97-413* H ✓
Info taken by: *Beth Isham, RN* Admit Date: *6/18/02*
Address: *66 Newton Street*
City: *Burlington* State: *VT* Zip: *05402*
Phone: *(802) 123-4567* Date of birth: *4/3/20*
Primary caregiver name & phone number: *husband (Dennis) (802) 123-4567*
Insurance name: *Medicare* Ins. #: *123-45-6789*
Is this a managed care policy (HMO)? *no*
Primary Dx: (Code *162.5*) *lung cancer* Date: *12/11/01*
(Code *877*) *pressure ulcer (coccyx)* Date: *3/13/02*
(Code *714.0*) *rheumatoid arthritis* Date: *1990s*
Procedures: (Code *86.28*) *decubitus care* Date: *6/1/02*
Referral source: *J. Silva. hospital SW* Phone: *555-765-2813*
Doctor name & phone #: *Frank Crabbe* Phone: *555-765-4321*
Doctor address: *9073 Parkway Drive, Burlington*
Hospital: *University Hospital* Admit: *6/1/02* Discharge: *6/16/02*
Functional limitations: Pain management, *nonambulatory, poor fine motor skills 2° rheumatoid arthritis*

Orders/Services: (specify amount, frequency and duration)
(SN:) *SN visits 3x/week & p.r.n. x 2 months*
(AL:) *CNA visits daily 5 days/week x 2 months*
(PT, OT) ST: *PT & OT evaluations and visits 2-3 x/week & p.r.n. x 2 months*
(MSW:) *MSW evaluation & weekly vs x 2 months*
Spiritual coordinator: *Rev. Carlson, St. Paul's Lutheran Church*
Counselor: *JoAnne Knowton, MSW*
Volunteer: *Rosalie Marshall – niece will provide care on weekends*
Other services provided: *shopping, laundry, meal prep*

Goals: *wound care, pain management, terminal care @ home*

Equipment: *needs commode, hospital bed, bedpan, Hoyer lift, side rail w/c*
Company & phone number: *Scott Medical Equipment (555) 765-9931*

Safety Measures: *side rails ↑* Nutritional req.: *diet as tolerated*

Functional limitations: (Circle applicable)
1. Amputation
2. Bowel/bladder
3. Contracture
4. Hearing
5. Paralysis
(6.) Endurance
(7.) Ambulation
8. Speech
9. Legally blind
A. Dyspnea with minimal exert
(B.) Other

Activities permitted: (Circle applicable)
1. Complete bedrest
2. Bedrest BRP
3. Up as tolerated
(4.) Transfer bed/chair
5. Partial wgt bearing
6. Independent at home
7. Crutches
8. Cane
(A.) Wheelchair
B. Walker
C. No restriction
D. Other - specify

Accessibility to bath: Y - (N) Shower: Y - (N) Bathroom: Y - (N) Exit: (Y) - N

Mental status: (Circle) Oriented Comatose Forgetful (Depressed) Disoriented Lethargic Agitated Other

- evidence that the home environment is safe for the procedure or treatment or can be safely adapted, and findings about the home and measures taken to ensure safe delivery of care
- rationale for treatment and patient response
- emergency and resource numbers given to the patient or caregiver (JCAHO requires that the patient or caregiver have 24-hour emergency telephone access to the agency or nurse)
- patient's or caregiver's ability to perform steps in home care procedures, including the patient's or caregiver's ability to perform return demonstration
- patient's or caregiver's ability to troubleshoot equipment, including a backup plan for a power failure
- patient's or caregiver's ability to recognize potential complications, respond appropriately, and get help when necessary.

DOCUMENTING PATIENT TEACHING

Correct documentation will help justify to your agency and to third-party payers your visits to teach the patient or caregiver. Find out about the patient's and his family's needs, resources, and support systems. This will help you outline the basic plan for teaching.

Remember that teaching is usually an ongoing process requiring more than one visit. Until the patient becomes independent, your documentation will help other nurses continue the teaching and identify additional areas of teaching. (See *Certification of instruction,* page 144.)

Keep a list of teaching and reference materials you have supplied to the patient or caregiver. Also, document modifications made to accommodate the patient's or caregiver's literacy skills and native language.

If the patient isn't physically or mentally able to perform the skills himself and no caregiver is available, report this in your documentation. The patient most likely isn't an appropriate candidate for home care. Never leave a patient alone to perform a procedure until he can express an understanding of it and perform it competently.

Be careful to call equipment by the same names used on the packages and in the teaching literature. Consider providing a glossary of terms and labeling machines to match your instructions. Make sure the patient can identify devices to eliminate confusion when speaking on the telephone. Document all teaching materials given to the patient, and keep copies of teaching materials in your records. You may want to videotape your instructions in the home if more than one caregiver will be providing care.

Most agencies require the patient to sign a teaching documentation record indicating that he accepts responsibility for learning self-care activities. This is a critical piece of documentation for the home care chart.

Home care forms

Key forms used to document home care include:

- agency assessment form and OASIS
- care plan
- progress notes
- nursing and discharge summaries
- Medicare-mandated forms.

CHART QUICK

Certification of instruction

The model patient-teaching form below shows what was taught to a home-care patient with an I.V. line. This type of form will help you document your teaching sessions clearly and completely.

CONTENT (check all that apply; fill in blanks as indicated)

1. ☐ Reason for therapy
2. Drug/Solution
   - ☐ Dose
   - ☐ Schedule
   - ☐ Label accuracy
   - ☐ Storage
   - ☐ Container integrity
3. Aseptic technique
   - ☐ Handwashing
   - ☐ Prepping caps/ connections
   - ☐ Tubing/cap/needs
   - ☐ Needleless adapter changes
4. Access device maintenance
   - Type/Name: ____________
   - ☑ Device / Site Inspection
   - ☐ Site care/Dsg. changes
   - ☐ Catheter clamping
   - ☑ Maintaining patency
     - ☑ Saline flushing
     - ☐ Heparin locking
     - ☐ Fdg. Tube /declogging
     - ☐ Self insertion of device
5. Drug preparation
   - ☑ Premixed containers
   - ☐ Compounding
   - ☐ Client additives
   - ☐ Piggyback lipids
6. Method of administration
   - ☐ Gravity
   - ☑ Pump (name): *IVAC pump*
   - ☐ Continuous
   - ☑ Intermittent
   - ☐ Cycle/Taper: ________
7. Administration technique
   - ☑ Pump rate/calibration
   - ☐ Priming tubing
   - ☐ Filter
   - ☐ Filling syringe
   - ☐ Loading pump
   - ☑ Access device hookup/disconnect
8. Potential complications/ Adverse effects
   - ☐ Patient drug information sheet reviewed ________
   - ☑ Pump alarms/ troubleshooting
   - ☑ Phlebitis/infiltration
   - ☐ Clotting/dislodgment
   - ☑ Infection
   - ☐ Air embolus
   - ☐ Breakage/cracking
   - ☐ Electrolyte imbalance
   - ☐ Fluid imbalance
   - ☐ Glucose intolerance
   - ☐ Aspiration
   - ☐ N / V / D / Cramping
   - ☐ Other: ____________
9. Self monitoring:
   - ☐ Weight ☑ Temperature
   - ☐ P ☐ PB
   - ☐ Urine S & A
     - ☐ Fingersticks
   - ☐ Other: ____________
10. Supply handling/disposal
    - ☑ Disposal of sharps/ supplies
    - ☐ Narcotics
    - ☑ Cleaning pump
    - ☐ Changing batteries
    - ☐ Blood/fluid precautions
    - ☐ Chemo/spill precautions
11. Information given to client re:
    - ☐ Pharmacy counseling
    - ☐ Advance directives
    - ☐ Inventory checks ______
    - ☑ Deliveries ________
    - ☑ 24-hour on-call staff ____
    - ☐ Reimbursement ______
    - ☐ Service complaints______
12. Safety/Disaster plan
    - ☑ Back up pump batteries _
    - ☐ Emergency room use ___
    - ☑ Electrical ________
    - ☐ Disaster________
    - ☑ Other: ________
13. Written instructions
    - ☑ Yes ☐ No If no why

☐ Client or caregiver demonstrates or verbalizes competency to perform home infusion therapy.

Comments: *Wife incorrectly changed pump battery. Procedure reviewed. Wife then demonstrated correct procedure. Wife also concerned about frequency of dressing changes. Access site nonreddened and not edematous. Protocol reviewed patient states he is satisfied to wait until scheduled dressing change tomorrow.*

Theory/Skill reviewed/Return demonstration completed:

Chris Banner, RN — *4-18-02*

Signature of RN Educator — Date

CERTIFICATION OF INSTRUCTION

I agree that I have been instructed as described above and understand that the above functions will be performed in the home by myself and caregiver, outside a hospital or medically supervised environment.

Robert Burns — *4-18-02*

Client/caregiver signature — Date

AGENCY ASSESSMENT FORM AND OASIS

When a patient is referred to your home care agency, you must complete a thorough and specific assessment and document the information on a patient assessment form.

Assess the patient's:

- physical status
- mental and emotional status
- home environment in relation to safety and support services
- knowledge of his disease or current condition, prognosis, and treatment plan
- potential for complying with the treatment plan.

Guidelines for use

As with any setting, be thorough during home care. A thorough patient assessment provides the information you need to plan appropriate care.

Consider the following:

- Obtain information about the patient's past and current health. Organize the interview by body system and ask open-ended questions.
- When taking a physical assessment, use a systematic approach, as is appropriate in any setting. For example, you may take a body-system or head-to-toe approach.
- When assessing the home environment, consider such factors as the presence of a caregiver, structural barriers, access to a telephone, and safety and hygiene practices.
- When assessing the patient's potential for complying with the treatment plan, consider such factors as history of psychiatric disorders, developmental status, substance abuse, comprehension, ability to read and write, and the presence of language barriers.
- OASIS isn't a substitute for a thorough assessment; it's an addition. Some agencies have integrated their assessment forms and OASIS. (See *Using the OASIS-B1 form,* pages 146 and 147.)
- OASIS guidelines specify the questions to be asked. All must be asked, even though the patient may decline to answer some. Note the ones he declines to answer on your record, and also report all responses and nonresponses to your supervisor.

CARE PLAN

Professional standards dictated by CHAP in 1993 — under the guidance of NLN — require you to develop a comprehensive care plan in cooperation with the patient and his caregivers.

In many aspects of care, the patient and his family become the decision makers. You must take this fact into account when developing your care plan; adjust your interventions, patient goals, and teaching accordingly. Also, take reimbursement into consideration.

Legally speaking, a care plan is the most direct evidence of your nursing judgment. If you outline a care plan and then deviate from it, a court may decide that you strayed from a reasonable standard of care. So be sure to update your care plan and make sure it fits the patient's needs.

Some agencies use the home care certification form and care plan form (required for Medicare reimbursement) as the official care plan for Medicare patients. Most home care agencies, however, require a separate care plan.

Agencies use a multidisciplinary, integrated care plan for those patients receiving more than one service, such as

(Text continues on page 149.)

CHART QUICK

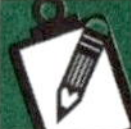

Using the OASIS-B1 form

The Oasis-B1 form includes more than 80 topics, such as socioeconomic, physiologic, and functional data; service utilization information; and mental, behavioral, and emotional data. The following is a portion of this form.

OUTCOME AND ASSESSMENT INFORMATION SET (OASIS-B1)

START OF CARE Assessment
(also used for Resumption of Care Following Inpatient Stay)

Client's Name: ______
Client Record No.: ______

Demographic/General Information

1. **(M0010)** Agency Medicare Provider Number: ______
2. **(M0012)** Agency Medicaid Provider Number: ______

Branch Identification
(Optional, for Agency Use)
3. **(M0014)** Branch State: ______
4. **(M0016)** Branch ID Number: ______
Agency-assigned

5. **(M0020)** Patient ID Number: QCB/811757
6. **(M0030)** Start of Care Date: 05 / 02 / 2002 (month / day / year)
7. **(M0032)** Resumption of Care Date: ___ / ___ / ___ (month / day / year)
   ☑ NA - Not Applicable
8. **(M0040)** Patient Name:
   Terry (First) S (MI)
   Elliot (Last) Mr. (Suffix)
   Patient Address:
   11 Second Street (Street, Route, Apt. Number)
   Hometown (City)
   (M0050) Patient State of Residence: PA
   (M0060) Patient Zip Code: 10981 - 1234
   Phone: (881) 555 - 2937
9. **(M0063)** Medicare Number: 134765482 A (including suffix)
   ☐ NA - No Medicare
10. **(M0064)** Social Security Number: 111 - 22 - 3333
    ☐ UK - Unknown or Not Available
11. **(M0065)** Medicaid Number: ______
    ☐ NA - No Medicaid
12. **(M0066)** Birth Date: 07 / 08 / 1926 (month / day / year)
13. **(M0069)** Gender:
    ☑ 1 - Male ☐ 2 - Female
14. **(M0072)** Primary Referring Physician ID: 222222 (UPIN#)
    ☐ UK - Unknown or Not Available
    Name Dr. Kyle Stevens
    Address 10 State Street
    Hometown, PA 10981
    Phone: (881) 555 - 6900
    Fax: (881) 555 - 6974
15. **(M0080)** Discipline of Person Completing Assessment:
    ☑ 1-RN ☐ 2-PT ☐ 3-SLP/ST ☐ 4-OT
16. **(M0090)** Date Assessment Completed: 05 / 02 / 2002 (month / day / year)
17. **(M0100)** This Assessment is Currently Being Completed for the Following Reason:
    Start/Resumption of Care
    ☑ 1 - Start of care – further visits planned
    ☐ 2 - Start of care – no further visits planned
    ☐ 3 - Resumption of care (after inpatient stay)

Using the OASIS-B1 form (continued)

Follow-Up
☐ 4 -Recertification (follow-up) reassessment [Go to M0150]
☐ 5 - Other follow-up [Go to M0150]
Transfer to an Inpatient Facility
☐ 6 - Transferred to an inpatient facility – patient not discharged from agency [Go to M0150]
☐ 7 - Transferred to an inpatient facility – patient discharged from agency [Go to M0150]
Discharge from Agency – Not to an Inpatient Facility
☐ 8 - Death at home [Go to M0150]
☐ 9 - Discharge from agency [Go to M0150]
☐ 10 - Discharge from agency – no visits completed after start/resumption of care assessment [Go to M0150]

18. Marital status:
☐ Not Married ☑ Married ☐ Widowed
☐ Divorced ☐ Separated ☐ Unknown

19. **(M0140)** Race/Ethnicity (as identified by patient):
(Mark all that apply.)
☐ 1 - American Indian or Alaska Native
☐ 2 - Asian
☐ 3 - Black or African-American
☐ 4 - Hispanic or Latino
☐ 5 - Native Hawaiian or Pacific Islander
☑ 6 - White
☐ UK - Unknown

20. Emergency contact:
Name *Susan Elliot*
Address *11 Second Street*
Hometown, PA 19081
Phone: (*881*) *555* - *2937*

21. **(M0150)** Current Payment Sources for Home Care:
(Mark all that apply.)
☐ 0 - None; no charge for current services
☑ 1 - Medicare (traditional fee-for-service)
☐ 2 - Medicare (HMO/managed care)
☐ 3 - Medicaid (traditional fee-for-service)
☐ 4 - Medicaid (HMO/managed care)
☐ 5 - Workers' compensation
☐ 6 - Title programs (e.g., Title III, V, or XX)
☐ 7 - Other government (e.g., CHAMPUS, VA, etc.)
☐ 8 - Private insurance
☐ 9 - Private HMO/managed care
☐ 10 - Self-pay
☐ 11 - Other (specify) ________
☐ UK - Unknown

22. **(M0160)** Financial Factors limiting the ability of the patient/family to meet basic health needs:
(Mark all that apply.)
☑ 0 - None
☐ 1 - Unable to afford medicine or medical supplies
☐ 2 - Unable to afford medical expenses that are not covered by insurance/Medicare (e.g., copayments)
☐ 3 - Unable to afford rent/utility bills
☐ 4 - Unable to afford food
☐ 5 - Other (specify) ________

Patient History

23. **(M0175)** From which of the following Inpatient Facilities was the patient discharged during the past 14 days?
(Mark all that apply.)
☐ 1 - Hospital
☐ 2 - Rehabilitation facility
☐ 3 - Skilled nursing facility
☐ 4 - Other nursing home
☐ 5 - Other (specify) ________
☑ NA - Patient was not discharged from an inpatient facility [If NA, go to M0200]

24. **(M0180)** Inpatient Discharge Date (most recent):
____ / ____ / ________
month day year
☐ UK - Unknown

CHART QUICK

Interdisciplinary care plan

The care plan is individualized for each patient. An example of this form is shown below.

Patient name: *Mary Lang*

Primary nurse: *N. Smith, RN*

Init. cert. period: ______

Recert period #1: ______

Recert period #2: ______

Problem	Goal	Approach	Initial Cert	Recert #1	Recert #2
Atrial fibrillation 2/6/02	*Maintain optimal cardiac output*	*1. Meds as ordered* *2. Monitor vs, inc. apical rhythm and rate* *3. observe for chest pain, dyspnea, palpitations, anxiety, etc.*	Goal Met? Y N Init: ____	Goal Met? Y N Init: ____	Goal Met? Y N Init: ____
Heart failure 5/21/02	*1. Maintain fluid and electrolyte balance* *2. Promote optimal gas exchange*	*1. Meds as ordered* *2. Nebulizer as ordered* *3. Draw labs as ordered* *4. I & O daily* *5. Monitor edema* *6. √ for SOB, dyspnea, congestion (lung sounds)* *7. amb. as tol* *8. semi Fowler's when sitting*	Goal Met? Y N Init: ____	Goal Met? Y N Init: ____	Goal Met? Y N Init: ____
Gastrostomy tube insertion 5/23/02	*1. Maintain optimal nutritional status* *2. Prevent skin breakdown*	*1. Magnacal 80 ml/hr* *2. Follow G-tube protocol, including site care & oral hygiene* *3. Weekly weights* *4. I&O daily* *5. √ for N/V, diarrhea*	Goal Met? Y N Init: ____	Goal Met? Y N Init: ____	Goal Met? Y N Init: ____

Intervention Codes *(please circle all that apply)*

A1. Skilled observation
A2. Foley insertion
A3. Bladder instillation
A4. Irrigation care (wd. dsg.)
A5. Irrigation decub. care - meds.
A6. Venipuncture
A7. Restorative nursing
A8. Postcataract care
A9. Bowel/Bladder training
A10. Chest physical (incl. postural drainage)
A11. Administer vit. B_{12}
A12. Prepare/Administer insulin
A13. Administer other
A14. Administer I.V.
A15. Teach ostomy care
A16. Teach nasogastric feeding
A17. Reposition nasogastric feeding tube
A18. Teach gastrostomy
A19. Teach parenteral nutrition
A20. Teach care of trach
A21. Administer care of trach
A22. Teach inhalation Rx
A23. Administer inhalation Rx
A24. Teach administration of injections
A25. Teach diabetic care
A26. Disimpaction/enema
A27. Other
Foot care (diabetic)
Teach diet
Teach disease process
Teach use of 0_2
Instruct re: Medication
child
A28. Wound care/dsg - closed
A29. Decubitus care - simple
A30. Teach care of indwelling catheter
A31. Management and evaluation of patient care plan
A32. Teaching and training (other)

physical or occupational therapy. (See *Interdisciplinary care plan.*)

Guidelines for use

To document most effectively on your care plan, follow these suggestions:

- Keep a copy of the care plan in the patient's home for easy reference by him and his family.
- Make sure the care plan is comprehensive by including more than the patient's physiologic problems. Also include documentation about the home environment, resources needed, and attitudes of the patient, family, and caregiver.
- Document physical changes that need to be made in the patient's home for him to receive proper care. Help the family find the resources to implement them.
- Describe the primary caregiver, including whether he lives with the patient, their relationship, his age and physical ability, and his willingness to help the patient. The patient's well-being may depend on this person's abilities.
- Show in your documentation how you made the most of the patient's strengths and resources. Strengths include support systems, good health habits and coping behaviors, a safe and healthful environment, and financial security. Resources include the physician, pharmacy, and medical equipment supplier.
- Continuously identify progress toward goals. If the patient can't make progress, discharge may be considered.
- If the patient is homebound, make sure this is documented at every visit and state the reason why. Medicare requires a patient receiving skilled home care to be homebound; however, some commercial insurers don't.
- Make sure that documentation reflects consistent adherence to the care plan by all caregivers. Have caregivers demonstrate the procedures they use for the care they provide, and document their skill level.
- Keep the record updated, noting changes in the patient's condition or care plan, and document when you report these changes to the physician. Medicare, Medicaid, and certain other third-party payers won't reimburse for skilled services not reported to the physician.
- Interdisciplinary care must be documented on an ongoing basis. Collaboration on patient care problems and changes to the care plan are described in detail on the patient's chart.

PROGRESS NOTES

The home care progress note, like notes in the acute care setting, is a place to document the patient's condition and significant events that occur while he's under your care. The progress note is written in chronological order based on each home visit.

Every time you visit a patient, you must write a progress note. These notes document:

- changes in the patient's condition
- skilled nursing interventions you performed related to the care plan
- patient's responses to the interventions
- events or incidents in the home that might affect the treatment plan
- patient's vital signs
- what you taught the patient and caregiver, including written instructional materials and brochures

- communication with other team members since the previous visit
- discharge plans
- time you arrived in the home and time you left the home.

Guidelines for use

The guidelines here will help you document safely and efficiently on progress notes:

- Document all events in chronological order.
- Avoid addendums.
- Provide a heading, such as "Nursing Progress Note," for each entry to identify your progress note because many members of the health care team use the progress notes.
- Use flow sheets and checklists to record vital signs, intake and output measurements, and nutritional data. Encourage the patient or caregiver to fill out these forms when appropriate. This gets them involved and increases their feeling of control.
- To help prevent the patient from feeling neglected, limit the time you spend documenting in the home. When possible, take time to complete your documenting while the patient sleeps or is otherwise occupied.
- Involve the patient in his own care and documentation by making statements like, "Here's what I've written about how your wound is healing. Is there anything else you want me to put in the notes?"
- If the patient has a medical emergency while you're there, accompany him to the hospital or emergency unit and stay until another caregiver takes over. Notify your supervisor, who will arrange coverage for your other patients, if necessary. Record all assessments and interventions performed until you're relieved. Note the date and time of transfer and the name of the caregiver who assumes responsibility.
- If documentation materials were completed and left in the patient's home, collect them at least once per week and take them to your home care agency. This keeps volumes of paper from piling up or becoming misplaced and also makes the records available for review by the agency supervisor.

NURSING AND DISCHARGE SUMMARIES

As a home health nurse, you must submit a regular patient progress report to the attending physician and the reimburser to confirm the need for continuing services. You must also complete a summary of the patient's progress and a discharge summary.

When writing a summary of the patient's progress, include:

- current problems, treatments, interventions, and instructions
- home care provided by other health care professionals, such as a physical therapist or speech pathologist
- reason for a change in services
- patient outcomes and responses — physical and emotional — to the services provided
- discharge plan.

Guidelines for use

You'll prepare a discharge summary to get the physician's approval to discharge a patient, to notify third-party payers that services have been terminated, and to officially close the case. The discharge summary also serves as a brief history for quick review if the patient is readmitted at a later date.

When writing these summaries, record:

- time frame covered
- services provided and names and titles of assigned staff
- third-party payer and whether the patient is eligible for future payment (he may have exhausted his annual benefits)
- clinical and psychosocial condition of the patient at discharge
- recommendations for further care
- caregiver involvement in care
- interruptions in home care such as readmissions to the hospital
- referrals to community agencies
- OASIS discharge information
- patient's response to and comprehension of patient-teaching efforts
- outcomes attained.

MEDICARE-MANDATED FORMS

CMS, the federal watchdog agency that oversees Medicare and Medicaid programs, requires home care agencies that receive Medicare funding to standardize their record keeping and documentation methods. Home care agencies must maintain the following forms for each qualified Medicare recipient:

- OASIS
- home care certification and care plan (see *Home care certification and care plan,* page 152)
- health update and patient information (see *Medical update and patient information,* page 153)
- notice of nondiscrimination.

In addition, home care nurses must document a physician's telephone orders. (See *Physician's telephone orders,* page 154.)

Medicare, through the fiscal intermediary, won't pay unless the required forms are properly completed, signed, and submitted. Forms are usually filled out by the nurse assigned to the patient, although some agencies have an admission team and a care team.

Future developments

Several major trends are emerging as the home care industry continues to evolve:

- More private insurers require preauthorization for home care services, which increases the paperwork burden for nurses.
- Fewer visits per episode of care are allowed. More focused reimbursement will dramatically alter the amount of home care patients will receive.
- The depth and breadth of federal regulations have placed increasing demands on care providers, and agencies will need to computerize record keeping.

Increased reliance on disease-specific management programs will eventually lead to the use of critical pathways that incorporate patient outcomes in home care. CMS and JCAHO are focused on outcomes. State departments of health services surveyors also have access to data. In addition, an agency's data are compared with data from similar agencies.

Increasingly, home health nurses are using laptop computers or handheld devices equipped with software designed to speed clinical documentation. Many of these programs are designed to help nurses develop a care plan, formulate goals, monitor patient progress, update medications, and generate visit notes.

This technology expedites the exchange of data between care providers and third-party payers. Nurses inexperienced in using computers should be

CHART QUICK

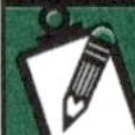

Home care certification and care plan

The form below is the official form for authorizing Medicare coverage for home care (also known as form 485). It includes space for assessing functional abilities and documenting care plan information.

Department of Health and Human Services
Health Care Financing Administration

Form Approved
OMB No. 0938-0357

HOME HEALTH CERTIFICATION AND PLAN OF CARE

1. Patient's HI Claim No.	2. Start Of Care Date	3. Certification Period	4. Medical Record No.	5. Provider No.
111-111	01/08/02	From: 03/08/02 To: 05/08/02	78-901	11-1213

6. Patient's Name and Address
Mary Lang
2218 Central Avenue
Wichita, Kansas

7. Provider's Name, Address and Telephone Number
Home Health Agency
301 Main St.
Wichita, Kansas

8. Date of Birth 10/04/29 9. Sex ☐ M ☑ F

		Date
11. ICD-9-CM 42731	Principal Diagnosis: atrial fibrillation	01/1/02
12. ICD-9-CM 0000	Surgical Procedure: gastrostomy tube insertion	03/3/02
13. ICD-9-CM 4280	Other Pertinent Diagnoses: heart failure	03/1/02
496	chr airway obstruct	11/29/01

10. Medications: Dose/Frequency/Route (N)ew (C)hanged
digoxin 0.125 mg P.O. q.d.; Lasix 20mg P.O. q.d.; warfarin 5mg P.O. q.d.; Capoten 12.5 mg b.i.d.; Proventil inh 2 puffs q.i.d./p.r.n.; MVI one P.O. q.d.; FeSO4 325 mg q.d.; Ex St Tylenol 500 mg q4h p.r.n.; albuterol 0.5cc with 3cc ns via nebulizer b.i.d.; 325 mg aspirin 1x daily.

14. DME and Supplies: gastrostomy tube supplies, cane

15. Safety Measures: prevent falls

16. Nutritional Req. magnacal 80ml/hr

17. Allergies: NKA

18.A. Functional Limitations
1 ☐ Amputation
2 ☐ Bowel/Bladder (Incontinence)
3 ☐ Contracture
4 ☐ Hearing
5 ☐ Paralysis
6 ☑ Endurance
7 ☐ Ambulation
8 ☐ Speech
9 ☐ Legally Blind
A ☐ Dyspnea With Minimal Exertion
B ☐ Other (Specify)

18.B. Activities Permitted
1 ☐ Complete Bedrest
2 ☐ Bedrest BRP
3 ☑ Up As Tolerated
4 ☐ Transfer Bed/Chair
5 ☐ Exercises Prescribed
6 ☐ Partial Weight Bearing
7 ☐ Independent At Home
8 ☐ Crutches
9 ☑ Cane
A ☐ Wheelchair
B ☐ Walker
C ☐ No Restrictions
D ☐ Other (Specify)

19. Mental Status: 1 ☑ Oriented 2 ☐ Comatose 3 ☐ Forgetful 4 ☐ Depressed 5 ☐ Disoriented 6 ☐ Lethargic 7 ☐ Agitated 8 ☐ Other

20. Prognosis: 1 ☐ Poor 2 ☐ Guarded 3 ☐ Fair 4 ☑ Good 5 ☐ Excellent

21. Orders for Discipline and Treatments (Specify Amount/Frequency/Duration)
RN: assess heart failure, effects of digoxin, monitor complaints of arthritis pain control; monitor gastrostomy tube site, help with gastrostomy feedings and tube care. Draw blood as ordered by MD. AID 2-3wk; assist with personal care and ADLs.

22. Goals/Rehabilitation Potential/Discharge Plans
Pt needs teaching reinforcement and emotional support for colostomy. Rehab potential is good. Skilled nursing facility.

23. Nurse's Signature and Date of Verbal SOC Where Applicable: N. Smith, RN 03/08/02

25. Date HHA Received Signed POT 03/08/02

24. Physician's Name and Address
M. Raser, MD
555 Main St.
Wichita, Kansas

26. I certify/recertify that this patient is confined to his/her home and needs intermittent skilled nursing care, physical therapy and/or speech therapy or continues to need occupational therapy. The patient is under my care, and I have authorized the services on this plan of care and will periodically review the plan.

27. Attending Physician's Signature and Date Signed
M. Raser, MD

28. Anyone who misrepresents, falsifies, or conceals essential information required for payment of Federal funds may be subject to fine, imprisonment, or civil penalty under applicable Federal laws.

Form HCFA-485 (C-4) (02-94) (Print Aligned) PROVIDER

CHART QUICK

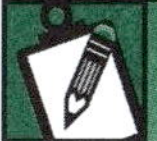

Medical update and patient information

To continue providing reimbursable skilled nursing care to a patient at home, Medicare requires you to complete the Medical Update and Patient Information form (also known as form 486).

Department of Health and Human Services
Health Care Financing Administration

Form Approved
OMB No. 0938-0357

MEDICAL UPDATE AND PATIENT INFORMATION

1. Patient's HI Claim No. 48-7850
2. SOC Date 01/08/02
3. Certification Period From: 06/08/02 To: 08/08/02
4. Medical Record No. 00-0000
5. Provider No. 98-7654
6. Patient's Name and Address James Dole, Main Street, Newark, NJ
7. Provider's Name Home Health Agency
8. Medicare Covered: [√] Y [ ] N
9. Date Physician Last Saw Patient: 03/07/02
10. Date Last Contacted Physician: 03/20/02
11. Is the Patient Receiving Care in an 1861 (J)(1) Skilled Nursing Facility or Equivalent? [ ] Y [√] N [ ] Do Not Know
12. [ ] Certification [ ] Recertification [ ] Modified
13. Dates of Last Inpatient Stay: Admission 06/01/02 Discharge 06/05/02
14. Type of Facility: A
15. Updated information: New Orders/Treatments/Clinical Facts/Summary from Each Discipline

Discipline	Visits (this bill)	Frequency and duration	Treatment codes	Total visits projected this cert.
SN	00	2MO2O3	AO1 AO6	07
ADL	00	3WKO9	FO4	27

SN A&O x 3. Skin warm, dry, pale, slight dyspnea noted with activity. Trace bilat. pedal edema, lungs clear. No complaints. Improved & increased feeling of well-being demonstrated. Peg tube patent and functioning well.
Correctly demonstrates checking for residual, peg tube site care.
AID pt seen 3x/wk. Increased difficulty ambulating. Expressed feelings of despair and hopelessness associated with physical condition.

16. Functional Limitations (Expand From 485 and Level of ADL) Reason Homebound/Prior Functional Status
Interaction between pt and daughter who wants pt to strive to live. Pt increasingly fearful of institutional care. Pt agrees to gastrostomy support group. CCSW to facilitate. Needs more encouragement to perform ADLs. Daughter more involved with care.
17. Supplementary Plan of Care on File from Physician Other than Referring Physician: (If Yes, Please Specify Giving Goals/Rehab. Potential/Discharge Plan) [ ] Y [ ] N
18. Unusual Home/Social Environment N/A
19. Indicate Any Time When the Home Health Agency Made a Visit and Patient was Not Home and Reason Why if Ascertainable
20. Specify Any Known Medical and/or Non-Medical Reasons the Patient Regularly Leaves Home and Frequency of Occurrence
21. Nurse or Therapist Completing or Reviewing Form M. Hoffner, RN
Date (Mo., Day, Yr.) 07/08/02

Form HCFA-486 (C3) (02-94) (Print Aligned)
PROVIDER

aware that documentation may take longer until they adjust to the new equipment.

New technology raises new concerns about confidentiality. For example, e-mail and faxes can easily end up in the wrong hands. When using either to

CHART QUICK

Physician's telephone orders

Home care nurses rely heavily on the use of telephone orders. The agency must follow guidelines established by the Centers for Medicare & Medicaid Services for taking and documenting these orders. Below is an example of a form used by one agency to fulfill documentation requirements. The order must be signed by the physician within 48 hours.

Facility name *Suburban Home Health Agency*		Address *123 Main Street*	
Last name *Smith*	First name *Kevin*	Attending doctor *Baker*	Admission no. *147-111-471*
Date ordered *05/22/02*	Date discontinued *05/25/02*	Orders *Tylenol 650 mg P.O. q6h p.r.n. Temp > 101°F*	
Signature of nurse receiving order *Mary Reo, RN*	Time *1820*	Signature of doctor	Date

transmit information about a patient, consider blacking out identifying data. Arrange for the recipient of a fax to wait at the other end for the fax to print.

Confidentiality when transmitting OASIS data on patients who aren't Medicare recipients continues to be a source of concern. Legislators and lawmakers will ultimately reconcile the parameters of government access to non-Medicare patients' clinical data.

In many cases, a home care agency will supply its nurses with laptop computers to streamline documentation. Laptop computers shouldn't be used by anyone other than agency personnel. You may be tempted to allow a computer-savvy spouse, friend, or child to add programs or manipulate data with all good intentions, but this is no more appropriate than it would be to let them read a patient's record. Finally, access to computer files should be protected by a password to prevent unauthorized individuals from entering files.

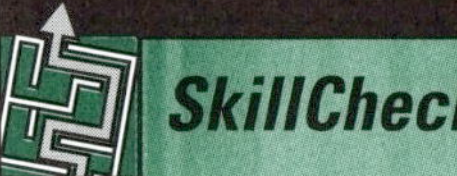

SkillCheck

1. All of the following have contributed to the growth of the home care industry except the:

a. development of a PPS system for home care agencies.

b. decreasing number of elderly patients.

c. use of OASIS.

d. increased availability of sophisticated home care equipment.

Answer: b. Because the number of patients of advanced age is increasing, the home care industry has responded with continued growth.

2. Home care agencies can expect a predetermined base payment for services from Medicare under which system?

a. OASIS
b. CHAP
c. JCAHO
d. PPS

Answer: d. PPS, or prospective payment system, was developed under the Balanced Budget Act of 1997 for Medicare home care services.

3. It's acceptable for you to skip questions when you are completing the OASIS-B1 form.

a. True
b. False

Answer: b. Every question on the OASIS-B1 form must be asked to the patient. If the patient chooses not to answer any question, this must be noted on the form.

4. What's one disadvantage of using new technology (for example, e-mail and fax) to transmit patient information?

a. It can be difficult to read.
b. It takes a long time to transmit.
c. It can put patient confidentiality at risk.
d. It requires duplicate documentation.

Answer: c. Because your transmittal could be seen or received by those for whom it isn't intended, try to arrange for the recipient of the fax to be waiting for the printout, or for both methods, consider blacking out identifying information.

5. Where should you document the patient's condition and significant events that may occur during your visit?

a. Care plan
b. OASIS
c. Flow sheet
d. Progress note

Answer: d. The progress note, written every time you visit a patient, is written in chronological order and should contain the patient's condition and significant events during the visit.

7 Documenting in special situations

Some situations require special types of documentation. These include certain legal situations and certain procedures you may be involved in or perform. This chapter explains these special situations, reviews your responsibilities, and provides guidelines to help you meet those responsibilities.

Legal situations

Every day, you face patient care situations that could land you in court. Being aware of these situations and knowing how to document them defensively can help you protect yourself.

INCIDENT REPORTS

Whenever you witness an adverse event, file an incident report. Some things to report are injuries from restraints, burns, or other causes; falls (even if the patient wasn't injured); and a patient's insistence on being discharged against medical advice. If an incident report form doesn't leave enough space to fully describe an incident, attach an additional page of comments. (See *Completing an incident report.*)

An incident report isn't part of the patient's chart, but it may be used later in litigation. The report has two functions:

- It informs the administration of the incident so the risk management staff can work on preventing similar incidents.
- It alerts the administration and the facility's insurance company to a potential claim and the need for further investigation.

Only people who witnessed an incident should fill out and sign an incident report, and each witness should file a separate report. Once the report is filed, it may be reviewed by the nursing supervisor, the physician who examined the patient after the incident, various department heads and administrators, the facility's attorney, and the insurance company.

Because incident reports will be read by many people and may even turn up in court, you must follow strict guidelines when completing them. (See *Tips for reporting incidents,* page 158.)

Facilities are continually revising their incident report forms; some have begun to use computerized forms. Incident reports are also processed by computer, which permits classifying and counting of incidents to indicate trends.

Documenting incidents in progress notes

When documenting an incident in the medical record, follow these guidelines:

CHART QUICK

Completing an incident report

When you witness a reportable event, you must fill out an incident report. Forms vary, but most include the following information.

INCIDENT REPORT

Name *Greta Manning*
Address *7 Worth Way, Boston, MA*
Phone *(617) 555-1122*

9 DATE OF INCIDENT	10 TIME OF INCIDENT
5/14/02	*1442*

11 EXACT LOCATION OF INCIDENT (Bldg., Floor, Room No., Area) *4 - Main, Rm 447*

Addressograph if patient

12 TYPE OF INCIDENT (CHECK ONE ONLY) ☐ PATIENT ☐ EMPLOYEE ☑ VISITOR ☐ VOLUNTEER ☐ OTHER (Specify)

13 DESCRIPTION OF THE INCIDENT (WHO, WHAT, WHEN, WHERE, HOW, WHY) (Use Back of Form if Necessary)

Wife of pt found on floor next to bed. States, "I was trying to put side rail down to sit on the bed and I fell down."

PATIENT FALL INCIDENTS

14 FLOOR CONDITIONS ☑ CLEAN & SMOOTH ☐ OTHER ☐ SLIPPERY (WET) — FRAME OF BED ☑ LOW ☐ HIGH — NIGHT LIGHT ☐ YES ☑ NO

15 WERE BED RAILS PRESENT? ☐ NO ☐ 1 UP ☐ 2 UP ☐ 3 UP ☐ 4 UP — 17 OTHER RESTRAINTS (TYPE & EXTENT)

18 AMBULATION PRIVILEGE ☐ UNLIMITED ☐ LIMITED WITH ASSISTANCE ☐ COMPLETE BEDREST ☐ OTHER

19 WAS NARCOTICS, ANALGESICS, HYPNOTICS, SEDATIVES, DIURETICS, ANTIHYPERTENSIVES OR ANTICONVULSANTS GIVEN DURING LAST 4 HOURS? ☑ YES ☐ NO
DRUG AMOUNT TIME

PATIENT INCIDENTS

20 PHYSICIAN NOTIFIED NAME OF PHYSICIAN *J. Reynolds, MD* DATE *5/14/02* TIME *1445* COMPLETE IF APPLICABLE

EMPLOYEE INCIDENTS

21 DEPARTMENT — 22 JOB TITLE — 23 SOCIAL SECURITY #
24 MARITAL STATUS

ALL INCIDENTS

27 SUPERVISOR NOTIFIED NAME OF SUPERVISOR *C. Jones, RN* DATE *5/14/02* TIME *1500* — 28 LOCATION (WHERE TREATMENT WAS RENDERED)

29 NAME, ADDRESS AND TELEPHONE NUMBER OF WITNESS(ES) OR PERSONS FAMILIAR WITH INCIDENT - WITNESS OR NOT
Connie Smith, RN (617) 555-0912 / Main Street, Boston, MA

30 SIGNATURE OF PERSON PREPARING REPORT *Connie Smith* — TITLE *RN* — 31. DATE OF REPORT *5/14/02*

PHYSICIAN'S REPORT - To be completed for all cases involving injury or illness (DO NOT USE ABBREVIATIONS) (Use back of Form if necessary)

DIAGNOSIS AND TREATMENT
Received patient in Emergency Department after reported fall in husband's room. 2 cm x 2 cm ecchymotic area noted on right hip. No broken skin integrity. No complaints of pain. X-rays negative for fracture. Good range of motion. Ice pack applied. ——— J. Reynolds, MD

33 DISPOSITION *sent home*

34 PERSON NOTIFIED OTHER THAN HOSPITAL PERSONNEL NAME AND ADDRESS *R. Manning (daughter) address same as pt* — 35 DATE *5/14/02* — 36 TIME *1500*

37 PHYSICIAN'S SIGNATURE *J. Reynolds, MD* — 38 DATE *5/14/02*

- Write a factual account of the incident, including treatment and follow-up care as well as the patient's response. This shows that the patient was closely monitored after the incident. Make sure the descriptions in the chart match those in the incident report.
- Don't write in your note that an incident report was completed. This destroys the confidential nature of the report and may result in a lawsuit. For the same reason, the physician should not write an order for an incident report in the chart.

CHECKLIST

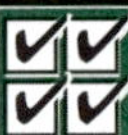

Tips for reporting incidents

In the past, a plaintiff's lawyer wasn't allowed to see incident reports. Today, however, many states allow lawyers access to incident reports if they make their requests through the proper channels. So when writing an incident report, keep in mind who may read it and follow these guidelines:

- ❑ Include essential information, such as the identity of the person involved in the incident, the exact time and place of the incident, and the name of the physician you notified.
- ❑ Document any unusual occurrences you witnessed.
- ❑ Record the events and the consequences for the patient in enough detail that administrators can decide whether to investigate further.
- ❑ Write objectively, avoiding opinions, judgments, conclusions, or assumptions about who or what caused the incident. Tell your opinions to your supervisor or the risk manager later.
- ❑ Describe only what you saw and heard along with the actions you took to provide care at the scene. Unless you saw a patient fall, write *Found pt lying on the floor.*
- ❑ Don't admit that you're at fault or blame someone else. Steer clear of statements such as *Better staffing would have prevented this incident.*
- ❑ Don't offer suggestions about how to prevent the incident from happening again.
- ❑ Don't include detailed statements from witnesses and descriptions of remedial action; these are normally part of an investigative follow-up.
- ❑ Don't put the report in the medical record. Send it to the person designated to review it according to your facility's policy.

▪ In documenting the incident, include everything the patient or family member says about his role in the incident. For example, you might write *Patient stated, "The nurse told me to ask for help before I went to the bathroom, but I decided to go on my own."* In a negligence lawsuit, this information may help the defense lawyer show that the incident was entirely or partially the patient's fault. If the jury finds that the patient was partially at fault, the concept of contributory negligence may be used to reduce or even eliminate the patient's recovery of damages.

INFORMED CONSENT

A patient must sign a consent form before most treatments and procedures. Informed consent means that he understands the proposed therapy and its risks and agrees to undergo it. The physician performing the procedure is legally responsible for explaining the procedure and its risks and obtaining consent. However, he may ask you to witness the patient's signature. Some facilities may specifically require that the person who informs the patient of the treatment or procedure be the one to obtain the consent. Check with your facility's legal counsel if you have any questions. (See *Witnessing a consent form.*)

CHECKLIST

Witnessing a consent form

After the physician informs the patient about a medical procedure, he may ask you to obtain the patient's signature on the consent form and then sign as a witness. Before doing this, review the checklist below.

- ❑ Make sure the patient is competent, awake, alert, and aware of what he's doing. He shouldn't be under the influence of alcohol, illicit drugs, or prescribed medications that impair his understanding or judgment.
- ❑ Ask the patient if the physician explained the diagnosis, proposed treatment, and expected outcome to his satisfaction. Also ask if he understands all that was said.
- ❑ Ask the patient if he has been told about the risks of the treatment or procedure, the possible consequences of refusing it, and alternative treatments or procedures.
- ❑ Ask the patient if he has concerns or questions about his condition or the treatment. If he does, help him get answers from the physician or other appropriate sources.
- ❑ Tell the patient that he can refuse the treatment without having other care or support withdrawn, and that he can withdraw his consent after giving it.
- ❑ Notify your nurse-manager and the physician immediately if you suspect that the patient has doubts about his condition or the procedure, hasn't been properly informed, or has been coerced into giving consent. Performing a procedure without voluntary consent may be considered battery.
- ❑ Objectively document your assessment of the patient's understanding in the chart, noting the situation, his responses, and actions you took.
- ❑ When you're satisfied that the patient is well informed, have him sign the consent form including the date and time, and then sign your name as a witness.
- ❑ Remember that you're responsible for obtaining oral informed consent for any procedures that you'll be performing, such as inserting an I.V. line or a urinary catheter, even though a general treatment consent was signed upon admission.

The legal requirement for obtaining informed consent can be waived in only two situations:

- if a mentally competent patient says that he doesn't want to know the details of a treatment or procedure
- if an urgent medical or surgical situation occurs. (Many facilities specify how you should document such an emergency.)

Most facilities use a standard consent form that lists the legal requirements for consent. If the patient doesn't understand the physician's explanation or asks for more information, answer all questions that fall within the scope of your practice. Be sure to document your interaction with the patient. (See *Informed consent,* page 160.)

ADVANCE DIRECTIVES

The Patient Self-Determination Act requires health care facilities to provide information about the patient's right to choose and refuse treatment. Facilities must also ask patients if they have ad-

CHART QUICK

Informed consent

If the patient signs a consent form, this implies that he understands the risks of a procedure and agrees to undergo it. Here's a typical form.

CONSENT FOR OPERATION AND RENDERING OF OTHER MEDICAL SERVICES

1. I hereby authorize Dr. *Wesley* to perform upon *Joseph Smith* (Patient name), the following surgical and/or medical procedures: (State specific nature of the procedures to be performed) *Exploratory laparotomy* .
2. I understand that the procedure(s) will be performed at Valley Medical Center by or under the supervision of Dr. *Wesley* , who is authorized to utilize the services of other doctors, or members of the house staff as he or she deems necessary or advisable.
3. It has been explained to me that during the course of the operation, unforeseen conditions may be revealed that necessitate an extension of the original procedure(s) or different procedure(s) than those set forth in Paragraph 1, I therefore authorize and request that the above named doctor, and his or her associates or assistants, perform such medical surgical procedures as are necessary and desirable in the exercise of professional judgment.
4. I understand the nature and purpose of the procedure(s), possible alternative methods of diagnosis or treatment, the risks involved, the possibility of complications, and the consequences of the procedure(s). I acknowledge that no guarantee or assurance has been made as to the results that may be obtained.
5. I authorize the above named doctor to administer local or regional anesthesia (for all other anesthesia management a separate consent must be signed by the patient or patient's authorized representative).
6. I understand that if it is necessary for me to receive a blood transfusion during this procedure or this hospitalization, the blood will be supplied by sources available to the hospital and tested in accordance with national and regional regulations. I understand that there are risks in transfusion, including but not limited to allergic, febrile, and hemolytic transfusion reactions, and the transmission of infectious diseases, such as hepatitis and AIDS (Acquired Immune Deficiency Syndrome). I hereby consent to blood transfusion(s) and blood derivative(s).
7. I hereby authorize representatives from Valley to photograph or videotape me for the purpose of research or medical education. It is understood and agreed that patient confidentiality shall be preserved.
8. I authorize the doctor named above and his or her associates and assistants and Valley Medical Center to preserve for scientific purposes or to dispose of any tissue, organs, or other body parts removed during surgery or other diagnostic procedures in accordance with customary medical practice.
9. I certify that I have read and fully understand the above consent statement. In addition, I have been afforded an opportunity to ask whatever questions I might have regarding the procedure(s) to be performed and they have been answered to my satisfaction.

Joseph Smith	*6/15/02*	*C. Gurney, RN*
Legal Patient or Authorized Representative (State Relationship to Patient)	Date	Witness

If the patient is unable to consent on his or her own behalf, complete the following:

Patient ______________ is unable to consent because ______________

Legally Responsible Person ______________ Doctor Obtaining Consent *M. Wesley, MD*

Tips for dealing with advance directives

Many patients wait until they're hospitalized to consider an advance directive or to make significant legal decisions. So be prepared to offer information and to record the patient's wishes in a legally appropriate manner. Here are some important points to remember.

Legal competence
Only a competent adult can execute a legally binding document. To prevent a patient's relatives from raising questions about his competence later, discuss his mental status with the physician and, possibly, a psychiatrist. Be sure to document his mental status assessment in the chart before he signs any legal document.

Living will and durable power of attorney
If a patient has a living will or durable power of attorney for health care, a copy should be in his chart. Also, you should know how to contact the person with decision-making power. If the patient doesn't have the document with him, ask a family member to bring it to the health care facility. As your patient's advocate, you must ensure that his wishes are properly executed. If conflicts arise, discuss them with your nurse-manager as well as with a risk manager.

If a patient wants to execute a living will during his hospital stay, you aren't required, or even allowed in some states, to sign as a witness. Many facilities have the social service or risk management department oversee this process. Find out who's responsible in your facility. The person who acts as witness can be held accountable for the patient's competence. Place the signed and witnessed document in the chart.

Last will and testament
In some facilities, dictating a patient's last will and testament is so commonplace that special forms have been designed for it. If this situation occurs often in your facility, discuss creating a form with your manager.

If no form exists in your facility, and a patient wants to dictate his last will and testament to you, document his request and what has been done to facilitate it, for example, who has been contacted and when.

If an administrator isn't available, two nurses should be present during dictation of the will. One should record the information in the chart, and both should sign it. In most instances, the patient's family will obtain their own legal representatives to process the recording of the will.

vance directives, which are documents that state a patient's wishes regarding life-sustaining medical care in case the patient is no longer able to indicate his own wishes. Your job is to document that the patient received the required information and whether he brought an advance directive with him. (See *Tips for dealing with advance directives*.)

When a patient's advance directive is given to the physician, the nurse's orders may change, depending on the patient's wishes. For example, if the patient's family submits an advance directive for a patient on life support who doesn't want to be kept alive on a ventilator, the patient may be removed from the ventilator and comfort measures provided.

The patient has the right to change advance directives at any time. Because the patient's requests may differ from what the family or physician wants, document discrepancies carefully. Use the social service or legal department for advice on how to proceed. (See *Advance directive checklist.*)

Common types of advance directives include:

- living will
- durable power of attorney for health care
- do-not-resuscitate (DNR) order.

Living will

In making a living will, a legally competent person declares what medical care he does or doesn't want if he develops a terminal illness. Living wills may apply only to treatment decisions made after a terminally ill patient becomes comatose and has no reasonable chance of recovery. They usually authorize the physician to withhold or discontinue lifesaving measures.

Most states recognize living wills as valid legal documents. Although the legal requirements vary from state to state, most states specify:

- circumstances under which a living will applies
- who is authorized to make a living will (usually only competent adults)
- limitations or restrictions on care that can be refused (for example, some states don't allow refusal of food and water)
- elements the living will must contain to be considered a legal document, including witnessing requirements
- who is immune from liability for following a living will's directions
- procedure for rescinding a living will.

Durable power of attorney

Durable power of attorney for health care enables a person to state what type of care he does or doesn't want. However, it also names another person to make health care choices if the patient becomes legally incompetent. This person is usually a family member or friend or, in rare instances, the physician.

DNR order

DNR orders are instructions not to attempt to resuscitate a patient who has suffered cardiac or respiratory failure. A DNR order may be appropriate if the patient has a terminal illness, is permanently unconscious, or won't respond to cardiopulmonary resuscitation (CPR). A terminally ill patient may ask not to be resuscitated if he experiences sudden cardiac arrest, or he may write this request into his advance directive.

If a patient asks not to be resuscitated, document his wishes and document his degree of awareness and orientation. Then contact your nurse-manager and request help from administration, legal services, or social services. Don't place yourself in the middle. Let the physician, patient, and his family make the decisions. If the physician knows about the patient's wish but still refuses to write a DNR order, document this in your notes. Like you, the physician must abide by the patient's wishes and may be found liable for negligence if he doesn't. If the patient has prepared an advance directive, make sure the physician has seen it.

If the patient doesn't ask for a DNR order, or if no policies exist, the physi-

CHART QUICK

Advance directive checklist

The Joint Commission on Accreditation of Healthcare Organizations requires that information on advance directives be charted on the admission assessment form. However, many facilities also use a checklist like the one shown below.

ADVANCE DIRECTIVE CHECKLIST

I. Distribution of Advance Directive Information

A. Advance directive information was presented to the patient: ☑

1. At the time of preadmission testing ☑
2. Upon inpatient admission ☐
3. Interpretive services contacted ☐
4. Information was read to the patient ☐

B. Advance directive information was presented to the next of kin as the patient is incapacitated ☐

C. Advance directive information was not distributed as the patient is incapacitated and no relative or next of kin was available ☐

RN: *Mary Barren, RN* Date: *6/15/02*

	Upon admission		Upon transfer to Critical Care Unit	
II. Assessment of Advance Directive upon admission	Yes	No	Yes	No
A. Does the patient have an advance directive?	☐	☑	☐	☐
If yes, was the attending physician notified?	☐	☐	☐	☐
B. If no advance directive, does the patient want to execute an advance directive?	☑	☐	☐	☐
If yes, was the attending physician notified?	☑	☐	☐	☐
Was the patient referred to resources?	☑	☐	☐	☐
RN	*Mary Barren, RN*			
Date	*6/15/02*			

III. Receipt of an Advance Directive after admission

A. The patient has presented an advance directive after admission and the attending physician has been notified.

RN ______ Date ______

cian may write the order if it's medically appropriate and the patient understands the impact of the DNR order. If the patient is incompetent, an appropriate surrogate must give consent for the physician to write the DNR order.

DNR orders should be reviewed periodically or whenever a significant

CHART QUICK

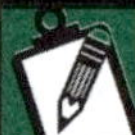

Witnessing refusal of treatment

To prevent misunderstandings and lawsuits if a patient refuses treatment, the physician must explain the risks involved in making this choice. If the patient still refuses treatment, the physician will ask him to sign a refusal-of-treatment release form, such as the one shown below, which you may need to witness.

REFUSAL-OF-TREATMENT RELEASE FORM

I, Joseph Arden, refuse to allow anyone to administer parenteral nutrition.

The risks attendant to my refusal have been fully explained to me, and I fully understand the benefits of this treatment. I also understand that my refusal of treatment seriously reduces my chances for regaining normal health and may endanger my life.

I hereby release Memorial General its nurses and employees, together with all physicians in any way connected with me as a patient, from liability for respecting and following my express wishes and direction.

Donna Burns
(Witness's signature)

Joseph Arden
(Patient's or legal guardian's signature)

6/05/02
(Date)

76
(Patient's age)

change occurs in the patient's clinical status.

PATIENTS WHO REFUSE TREATMENT

You're also responsible for helping patients make informed decisions about continuing treatment. When treatment is refused, important patient care, safety, and documentation issues come into play.

Refusing treatment

A mentally competent adult can legally refuse treatment if he has been fully informed about his medical condition and the likely consequences of his refusal. This means he can refuse mechanical ventilation, tube feedings, antibiotics, fluids, and other treatments that are needed to keep him alive.

When your patient refuses treatment, document his exact words. Inform him of the risks involved in refusing treatment, preferably in writing. If he still refuses treatment, document that you didn't provide the prescribed treatment, and then notify the physician. The physician will explain the risks to the patient again. If he continues to refuse treatment, the physician will ask him to sign a refusal-of-treatment release form, which you may need to sign as a witness. (See *Witnessing refusal of treatment.*)

If the patient won't sign this form, document this fact, too. For extra protection, your facility may require you to have the patient's spouse or closest relative sign another refusal-of-treatment release form.

More and more facilities are informing patients soon after admission about their future treatment options. Discuss the patient's wishes at your first opportunity, and document the discussion in case he becomes incompetent later. It may be helpful to use a chaplain or social services worker to speak with the patient to verify his wishes.

Legal guidelines

Failure to respond appropriately to a patient's refusal to accept treatment may have serious legal consequences. To prevent problems, take these steps:

- Confirm the patient's condition and prognosis with the physician and record them in the medical record.
- Make sure the physician documented the patient's understanding of the consequences of his refusal, such as pain or decreased life expectancy or quality of life.
- Search the medical record for a living will, durable power of attorney for health care, or letters from people who heard the patient express his wishes.
- Search the medical record for documentation of conversations between the patient and health care providers, including the conversation about the patient's final decision to withhold treatment. Documentation should include the dates of conversations, the full names of people involved, the circumstances, and what treatments and medical conditions were discussed.
- DNR orders should be reviewed every 48 to 72 hours, or according to your facility's policy.
- DNR orders must be written; they can't be provided as verbal orders or telephone orders.
- Refuse written or spoken orders for "slow codes." They may specify calling the physician before resuscitating a patient, doing CPR but withholding drugs, giving oxygen but withholding CPR, or not putting a patient on a ventilator. These orders are unethical and illegal.
- Suggest that your facility set up an ethics committee to resolve problems about withholding treatment.

DOCUMENTING FOR UNLICENSED PERSONNEL

Anyone reading your notes assumes these notes are a firsthand account of care provided — unless you document otherwise. In some settings, nursing assistants and technicians aren't allowed to make formal chart entries. In such a case, determine what care was provided, assess the patient and the task performed (for example, a dressing change), and document your findings. Be sure to record the full names and titles of unlicensed personnel who provided care. Don't just record their initials.

If your facility allows unlicensed personnel to document, you may have to countersign their notes. If your facility's policy states that the person must provide care in your presence, don't countersign unless you actually witness her actions. If the policy says that you don't have to be there, your countersigning indicates that the notes describe care that other people had the authority and competence to perform and that you verified that the procedures were performed. You can specifically document that you reviewed the notes and consulted with the technician on certain aspects of care. Of course,

CHART QUICK

Physical restraint order

A form, such as the one shown below, must be in the patient's chart before physical restraints are applied.

Date: 6/25/02 Time: 0315

Reason for restraint use (circle all that apply):

1. High risk of self-harm
2. High risk of harm to others
3. High risk of removing tubes, equipment, invasive lines Ⓡ subclavian CV line
4. High risk of causing significant disruption of the treatment environment
5. Other ______

Duration of restraint (Not to exceed 24 hr): 24

Type of restraint (circle all that apply):

Vest	
(Left mitt)	(Right mitt)
Left wrist	Right wrist
Left ankle	Right ankle
Other ______	

Physician's signature J. Donnelly, MD

you must document any follow-up care you provide.

USING RESTRAINTS

When physical restraints are ordered for a patient, your job is to check the patient frequently for problems associated with the restraints, perform range-of-motion exercises on all extremities, and then document your care. Most facilities have a policy outlining the proper procedure for using restraints. You may also recommend to the physician that he order physical restraints for a patient and document your observations in the progress notes. The physician must reevaluate the need for physical restraints and rewrite orders for them every 24 hours. (See *Physical restraint order*.)

If a competent patient refuses physical restraints, a facility may require him to sign a release absolving everyone involved of liability if he's injured as a result.

PATIENTS WHO REQUEST TO SEE THEIR CHARTS

A patient has a legal right to read his medical record. He may ask to see it because he's confused about the care he's receiving. First, ask him if he has questions about his treatment, and try to clear up any confusion.

If he still wants to see the record, check your facility's policy to see whether he has to read it in your presence. Document questions the patient asks about the record or statements he makes about it as well as what you say to him.

Never release medical records to unauthorized people, including family members and police officers. Refer all requests from insurance companies to the appropriate administrator, and refer other requests to your nurse-manager. Be sure to notify your nurse-manager if you have doubts about the validity of a request — she may want to notify the facility's administrator.

PATIENTS WHO LEAVE AGAINST MEDICAL ADVICE

The law says that a mentally competent patient can leave a facility at any time. Having the patient sign an against-medical-advice (AMA) form protects you, the physicians, and the facility if problems arise from his unapproved discharge.

The AMA form should clearly document that the patient knows he's leaving against medical advice, that he has been advised of and understands the risks of leaving, and that he knows he can come back. Use his own words to describe his refusal.

Here's what to include on the AMA form:

- names of relatives or friends notified of the patient's decision and the dates and times of the notifications
- explanation of the risks and consequences of the AMA discharge, as told to the patient, and the name of the person who provided the explanation
- other places the patient can go for follow-up care
- names of people accompanying the patient at discharge and the instructions given to them
- patient's destination after discharge.

If the patient leaves without anyone's knowledge or if he refuses to sign the AMA form, check your facility's policy; you most likely have to fill out an incident report in either situation.

In the progress notes, document statements and actions that reflect the patient's mental state at the time he left your facility. This helps protect you, the physician, security, and the facility against a charge of negligence if the patient later claims that he was mentally incompetent at the time of discharge and was improperly supervised while in that state.

Suppose a patient never says anything about leaving, but on rounds you discover he's missing? If you can't find him in the facility, notify your nurse-manager and the physician; then try to contact the patient's home. If he isn't there, call the police if you think the patient might hurt himself or others, especially if he left the hospital with any medical devices.

Document the time you discovered the patient missing, your attempts to find him, the people you notified, and other pertinent information.

Procedures

You'll need to document the procedures you perform, the procedures you assist the physician in performing, and various others. Following are guidelines to help you document completely in these situations.

GUIDELINES FOR DOCUMENTING NURSING PROCEDURES

Your notes about routine nursing procedures usually appear in the patient's chart, on flow sheets, or on graphic forms. Whatever your health care facility's requirements are, you need to include this information in your documentation:

- what procedure was performed
- when it was performed
- who performed it
- how it was performed
- how well the patient tolerated it
- adverse reactions to the procedure, if any.

The following section outlines information that must be documented for several nursing procedures.

DRUG ADMINISTRATION

A medication administration record (MAR) is part of most documentation systems. It may be included in the medication Kardex, or it may be on a separate sheet. In either case, it's the central record of medication orders and their execution and is part of the patient's permanent record.

When documenting on the MAR, follow these guidelines:

- Follow your facility's policies and procedures for recording drug orders and administration.
- Record the patient's full name, medical record number, and allergy information on each MAR.
- Immediately document the drug's name, dose, route of administration, and frequency; the number of doses ordered or the stop date (if applicable); and the administration time for doses given.
- Write legibly.
- Use only standard abbreviations. When in doubt, write out the word or phrase.
- After administering the first dose, sign your full name, licensure status, and initials in the appropriate space.
- Record drug administration immediately so that another nurse doesn't inadvertently repeat the dose.
- If you chart by computer, do so right after giving each drug—especially if you don't use printouts as a backup. This gives all team members access to the latest drug administration data.
- If a specific assessment parameter must be monitored during drug administration, document this requirement on the MAR. For example, when digoxin is administered, the patient's pulse rate needs to be monitored and documented on the MAR.
- If you didn't give a drug, circle the time and document the reason for the omission.
- If you suspect that a patient's illness, injury, or death was drug-related, report this to the pharmacy department, who will relay the information to the Food and Drug Administration.

As-needed medications

Document all as-needed drugs when administered, including reason for giving and the patient's response. For specific drugs given as needed, follow these guidelines:

- For eyedrops, eardrops, or nose drops, document the number instilled as well as the administration route.
- For suppositories, document the type (rectal, vaginal, or urethral) and how the patient tolerated it.
- For dermal drugs, document the size and location of the area where you ap-

plied the drug and the condition of the skin or wound.

- For dermal patches, document the location of the patch.
- For I.V., I.M., or subcutaneous medications, document the dose given and the location of administration.

If you administer as-needed drugs according to accepted standards, you don't need to document more specific information. However, if your MAR doesn't have space to document, for example, a patient's response to a drug or refusal to take a drug, document that information in the progress notes.

Drug abuse or refusal

If the patient refuses or abuses medications, describe the event in his chart. Here are some situations needing careful documentation:

- You discover nonprescribed drugs at the patient's bedside. Document the type of medication (pill or powder), the amount of medication, and its color and shape. (You may wish to send the drug to the pharmacy for identification.) Follow your facility's policy regarding the completion of an appropriate report.
- You find a supply of prescribed drugs in the patient's bedside table, indicating that he isn't taking each dose. Record the type and amount of medication.
- You notice a sudden change in the patient's behavior after he has visitors, and you suspect them of giving him narcotics or other drugs. Document how the patient appeared before the visitors came and afterward. Notify the physician immediately and follow your facility's policy.
- You offer prescribed medications and the patient refuses to take them. Document the refusal, the reason for it (if he tells you), and the medication. This prevents the refusal from being misinterpreted as an omission or a medication error on your part. An example of this is *Pt refused K-Dur tabs, stating that "they were too big and make me feel like I am choking when I try to swallow them."*

Report medication abuse or refusal to the physician. When you do so, document the name of the physician and the date and time of notification.

Narcotic administration

Whenever you give a narcotic, you must document it according to federal, state, and facility regulations. These regulations require you to:

- sign out the drug on the appropriate form
- verify the amount of drug in the container before giving it
- have another nurse document your activity and observe you if you must waste or discard part of a narcotic dose
- count narcotics after each shift.

Two nurses should be present to count narcotic drugs — preferably the oncoming and off-going nurse. If you discover a discrepancy in the narcotic count, report it, following your facility's policy. Also, file an incident report. An investigation will follow.

I.V. THERAPY

More than 80% of hospitalized patients receive some form of I.V. therapy, such as fluid or electrolyte replacement, total parenteral nutrition (TPN), drugs, or blood products. Document all facets of I.V. therapy carefully, including subsequent complications. Your facility may have you document in the progress notes, on a special I.V. therapy sheet or in a flowchart, or in another format.

After establishing an I.V. route, document:
- date, time, and venipuncture site
- equipment used, such as the type and gauge of the catheter or needle
- number of venipuncture attempts made and the type of assistance required (if applicable).

Once per shift, document:
- type, amount, and flow rate of I.V. fluid
- condition of the I.V. site
- that you flushed the I.V. line as well as what medication you used.

Update your records each time you change the insertion site, venipuncture device, or I.V. tubing. Also, document the reason you changed the I.V. site, such as extravasation, phlebitis, occlusion, patient removal, or a routine change.

Document complications precisely. For example, record if extravasation occurs and what interventions you took, such as stopping the I.V. infusion, assessing the amount of fluid infiltrated, and notifying the physician.

If a chemotherapeutic drug extravasates, stop the I.V. infusion immediately and follow the procedure specified by your health care facility. Document the appearance of the I.V. site, the treatment you gave (especially antidotes), and the type of dressing you applied. Document the amount of discarded medication.

If the patient has an allergic reaction during I.V. therapy, stop the infusion and notify the physician immediately. Then document all pertinent information about the reaction as well as your interventions and the patient's response.

Last, record patient and family teaching, such as explaining the purpose of I.V. therapy, describing the procedure itself, and discussing possible complications.

TPN

If a patient is receiving TPN, document:
- type and location of the central line
- condition of the insertion site
- volume and rate of the solution infused.

When you discontinue a central or peripheral I.V. line for TPN, record:
- date and time
- type of dressing applied
- appearance of the administration site.

Blood transfusions

Whenever you administer blood or blood components — such as packed cells, plasma, platelets, or cryoprecipitates — use proper identification and crossmatching procedures. Also, check the expiration date of the product and clearly document that you matched the label on the blood bag to:
- patient's name
- patient's medical record number
- patient's blood group or type
- patient's and donor's Rh factor
- crossmatch data
- blood bank identification number.

In addition, the blood or blood component must be identified by two health care professionals, both of whom sign the slip that comes with the blood and verify that the information is correct.

Once you determine that the information on the blood bag label is correct, you may administer the transfusion. On the transfusion record, document:
- dates and times the transfusion was started and completed

CHART QUICK

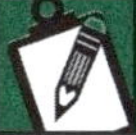

Documenting a blood transfusion reaction

The sample progress note shown below is an example of how to document a blood transfusion reaction.

Date	Time	Sign entries
6/19/02	1130	Pt reports nausea and chills. PRBC transfusion started at 1030 hr.
		Cyanosis of the lips noted at 1100 hr with first unit of PRBCs transfus-
		ing. Stopped infusion. Approximately 100 ml infused. Tubing changed.
		I.V. of 1,000 ml NSS infusing at 40 ml/hr in left hand. Dr. Dunn noti-
		fied. BP 170/90; P 110; R 28; T 99.4° F. Blood sample taken from PRBCs.
		Remaining blood discarded. Two red-top tubes of blood drawn from pt
		and sent to lab. Urine specimen obtained and sent to lab for UA. Pt
		given diphenhydramine 50 mg I.M. Two blankets placed on pt. ———
		——— Anne Grasso, RN
	1145	Pt reports he's getting warmer and less nauseated. BP 164/86; P 100; R
		24; T 99.2° F. ——— Anne Grosso, RN
	1200	Pt without chills or nausea. I.V. 1,000 ml NSS infusing at 80 ml/hr in
		left hand. BP 156/82; P 92; R 22; T 98.9°F. ——— Anne Grasso, RN

- name of the health care professional who verified the information
- type and gauge of the catheter used
- total amount of the transfusion
- patient's vital signs before, during, and after the transfusion
- infusion device used, if any, and its flow rate
- blood warming unit used, if any.

If the patient receives his own blood, document the amount retrieved and reinfused in the intake and output records. Document the results of laboratory tests performed during and after the autotransfusion, paying special attention to the coagulation profile, hematocrit, and arterial blood gas (ABG), hemoglobin, and calcium levels. Also document the patient's pretransfusion and posttransfusion vital signs.

If the patient develops a transfusion reaction, stop the transfusion immediately and notify the physician. On a transfusion reaction form or in the progress notes, document:

- time and date of the reaction
- type and amount of infused blood or blood products
- times you started and stopped the transfusion
- clinical signs in order of occurrence
- patient's vital signs per facility protocol
- whether urine specimens and blood samples were sent to the laboratory for analysis
- treatment you gave and the patient's response to it.

You may need to send the noninfused blood and tubing back to the blood bank. Follow your facility policy. (See *Documenting a blood transfusion reaction.*)

CHECKLIST

Documenting postsurgical status

When your patient recovers from anesthesia, he'll be transferred from the postanesthesia care unit (PACU) to his assigned unit for ongoing recovery and care. As his nurse, you're responsible for the four-part document that travels with him. Make sure the OR-PACU report is complete by checking for the following information.

Part 1: History
This section of the report should describe the patient's pertinent medical and surgical history, including drug allergies, medication history, chronic illnesses, significant surgical history, hospitalizations, and smoking history.

Part 2: Operation
This section describes the surgery itself and should include:
- ❑ procedure performed
- ❑ type and dosage of anesthetics
- ❑ how long the patient was anesthetized
- ❑ patient's vital signs throughout surgery
- ❑ volume of fluid lost and replaced
- ❑ drugs administered
- ❑ surgical complications
- ❑ tourniquet time
- ❑ drains, tubes, implants, or dressings used during surgery and removed or still in place.

Part 3: Postanesthesia period
This part of the record includes information about:
- ❑ pain medications and pain control devices the patient received and how he responded to them
- ❑ interventions that should continue on the unit, such as frequent circulatory, motor, and neurologic checks if the patient underwent leg surgery and had a tourniquet on for a long time
- ❑ a flow sheet showing the patient's postanesthesia recovery scores on arrival and discharge in the areas of activity level, respiration, circulation, and level of consciousness (LOC)
- ❑ unusual events or complications that occurred in the PACU; for example, nausea or vomiting, shivering, hypothermia, arrhythmias, central anticholinergic syndrome, sore throat, back or neck pain, corneal abrasion, tooth loss during intubation, swollen lips or tongue, pharyngeal or laryngeal abrasion, and postspinal headache.

Part 4: Current status
This section should describe the patient's status at the time of transfer back to the unit. Information should include his vital signs, LOC, sensorium, and the condition of the surgical site.

SURGICAL INCISION CARE

When a patient returns from surgery, document his vital signs and level of consciousness (LOC) and carefully record information about his surgical incision, drains, and the care you provide.

Study the records that travel with the patient from the postanesthesia care unit. (See *Documenting postsurgical status.*)

Look for a physician's order stating whether you or he will perform the first dressing change. If you'll be performing it, document:

- type of wound care performed
- wound appearance (size, color, condition of margins, presence of wound closure devices, and necrotic tissue); odor, if any; location of drains; and drainage characteristics (type, color, consistency, and amount)
- type and amount of dressing and whether a pouch was applied
- additional wound care procedures, such as drain management, irrigation and packing, or application of a topical medication
- how the patient tolerated the dressing change
- teaching provided to the patient (or family, if applicable).

Document special or detailed wound care instructions and pain management measures on the nursing care plan. Also document the color and amount of measurable drainage on the intake and output form.

If the patient needs wound care after discharge, provide patient teaching and document it. Document that you explained aseptic technique, described how to examine the wound for infection or other complications, demonstrated how to change the dressing, and gave written instructions for home care. Also document whether the patient demonstrates an understanding of the instructions and can perform wound care measures.

PACEMAKER CARE

If the patient has a temporary pacemaker inserted, record:

- date and time of placement
- reason for placement
- pacemaker settings
- patient's response
- patient's LOC and vital signs, including which arm you used to obtain the blood pressure reading
- complications, such as chest pain or signs of infection
- interventions, such as X-ray studies, to verify correct electrode placement
- medications that may have been given before or during the procedure.

Make sure the rhythm strip includes the patient's name and the date and time of placement.

If the patient has a transcutaneous pacemaker, document the reason for this type of pacing, the time pacing started, and the locations of the electrodes.

Document the information obtained from a 12-lead electrocardiogram (ECG). Place rhythm strips in the medical record before, during, and after pacemaker placement; any time pacemaker settings change; and any time the patient receives treatment for a pacemaker complication.

As ECG monitoring continues, record capture, sensing rate, intrinsic beats, and competition of paced and intrinsic rhythms.

PERITONEAL DIALYSIS

If your patient is receiving peritoneal dialysis, monitor and document his response to treatment during and after the procedure. Be sure to document:

- vital signs per facility protocol
- abrupt changes in the patient's condition and your notification of the physician
- amount of dialysate infused and drained and medications added (Complete a dialysis flowchart every 24 hours.)
- effluent's characteristics (color and clarity) and the assessed negative or

positive fluid balance at the end of each infusion-dwell-drain cycle

- patient's daily weight (immediately after the drain phase) and abdominal girth, noting the time of day and variations in the weighing and measuring technique
- physical assessment findings
- fluid status
- equipment problems, such as kinked tubing or mechanical malfunction, and your interventions
- condition of the patient's skin at the catheter site
- patient's reports of unusual discomfort or pain and your interventions
- any break in aseptic technique and notification of the physician
- whether the patient or a family member performs the peritoneal dialysis procedure.

PERITONEAL LAVAGE

For the patient recovering from peritoneal lavage, document:

- vital signs and symptoms of shock, such as tachycardia, decreased blood pressure, diaphoresis, dyspnea, or vertigo
- condition of the incision site
- type and size of the peritoneal dialysis catheter used
- type and amount of solution instilled into the peritoneal cavity
- amount and color of the fluid withdrawn from the peritoneal cavity and whether it flowed freely in and out
- what specimens were obtained and sent to the laboratory for analysis
- complications that occurred and your interventions.

THORACIC DRAINAGE

If your patient has thoracic drainage, initially record:

- date and time the drainage began
- type of system used
- amount of suction applied to the pleural cavity
- presence or absence of bubbling or fluctuation in the water-seal chamber
- amount and type of drainage
- patient's respiratory status.

At the end of each shift, record the following information:

- how frequently you inspected the drainage system
- presence or absence of bubbling or fluctuation in the water-seal chamber
- patient's respiratory status
- condition of the chest dressings
- type, amount, and route of pain medication you gave
- complications and subsequent interventions.

Ongoing documentation should include:

- color, consistency, and amount of thoracic drainage in the collection chamber as well as the time and date of each observation
- patient-teaching sessions and activities you taught the patient to perform, such as coughing and deep-breathing exercises, sitting upright, and splinting the insertion site to minimize pain
- rate and quality of the patient's respirations and your auscultation findings
- complications, such as cyanosis, rapid or shallow breathing, subcutaneous emphysema, chest pain, or excessive bleeding, and the time and date you notified the physician
- dressing changes and the patient's skin condition at the chest tube insertion site.

CARDIAC MONITORING

For the patient receiving cardiac monitoring, include in your notes:

- date and time the monitoring began
- monitoring leads used
- rhythm strip readings labeled with the patient's name and room number and the date and time
- changes in the patient's condition.

If the patient is to continue cardiac monitoring after discharge, document:

- which caregivers can interpret dangerous rhythms and perform CPR
- patient and family teaching, including troubleshooting techniques to use if the monitor malfunctions
- referrals to equipment suppliers, home care agencies, and other community resources.

CHEST PHYSIOTHERAPY

Whenever you perform chest physiotherapy, document:

- date and time of your interventions
- patient's positions for secretion drainage and how long he remains in each
- chest segments you percussed or vibrated
- characteristics of the secretion expelled, including color, amount, odor, viscosity, and the presence of blood
- patient's tolerance of the chest physiotherapy
- complications and your interventions.

MECHANICAL VENTILATION

For patients receiving mechanical ventilation, initially document:

- date and time the mechanical ventilation began
- type of ventilator used and its settings
- patient's responses to mechanical ventilation, including vital signs, breath sounds, use of accessory muscles, secretions, intake and output, and weight.

Throughout mechanical ventilation, document:

- complications and subsequent interventions
- pertinent laboratory data, including results of ABG analysis and oxygen saturation findings
- duration of spontaneous breathing and the ability to maintain the weaning schedule for patients receiving pressure support ventilation or those using a T-piece or tracheostomy collar
- rate of controlled breaths, the time of each breath rate reduction, and the rate of spontaneous respirations for patients receiving intermittent mandatory ventilation, with or without pressure support ventilation
- adjustments made in ventilator settings as a result of ABG levels
- adjustments of ventilator components, such as draining condensate into a collection trap and changing, cleaning, or discarding the tubing
- interventions to increase mobility, protect skin integrity, or enhance ventilation; for example, active or passive range-of-motion exercises, turning, or positioning the patient upright for lung expansion
- presence and characteristics of secretions
- type and frequency of oral care provided
- assessment findings related to LOC, peripheral circulation, urine output, decreased cardiac output, fluid volume excess, or dehydration
- patient's sleep and wake periods, noting significant trends
- patient and family teaching in preparation for the patient's discharge, especially that associated with ventilator care and settings, artificial airway care,

CHART QUICK

Documenting NG tube insertion

The sample progress note shown below is an example of how to document a nasogastric (NG) tube insertion procedure.

Date	Time	Sign entries
4/30/02	2100	#12 Fr. NG tube placed in Ⓡ nare. Placement verified via auscultation
		and X-ray. Tube attached to low intermittent suction as ordered.
		Drainage dark brown; heme +. Dr. Cohen notified. Hypoactive bowel sounds
		in all 4 quadrants. Pt tolerated procedure well.———Diane Harris, RN

communication, nutrition, and therapeutic exercise

- teaching discussions and demonstrations related to signs and symptoms of infection and equipment functioning
- referrals to equipment vendors, home care agencies, and other community resources.

NASOGASTRIC TUBE INSERTION AND REMOVAL

After you insert a nasogastric (NG) tube, record:

- type and size of the NG tube
- date, time, and insertion route (left naris, right naris, mouth)
- type and amount of suction
- amount, color, consistency, and odor of the drainage
- how the patient tolerated the insertion procedure
- signs and symptoms of complications, such as nausea, vomiting, and abdominal distention
- method of placement verification (for example, auscultation of air in gastric cavity or X-ray)
- subsequent irrigation procedures and problems occurring afterward, if any.

Record information about irrigations on an input and output sheet. (See *Documenting NG tube insertion.*)

After you remove an NG tube, record:

- date and time of removal
- how the patient tolerated the procedure
- unusual events accompanying tube removal, such as nausea, vomiting, abdominal distention, and food intolerance.

SEIZURE MANAGEMENT

If your patient had a seizure while hospitalized, document:

- what seizure precautions you took
- date and time the seizure began and its duration
- precipitating factors, including aura-like sensations reported by the patient
- involuntary behavior occurring before the seizure, such as lip smacking, chewing movements, or hand and eye movements
- incontinence during the seizure
- patient's vital signs (response to the seizure)
- what medications you gave

- complications resulting from the medications or the seizure and your interventions
- your assessment of the patient's post-seizure mental status
- what and when you reported to the physician.

SUTURE AND STAPLE REMOVAL

If the physician writes an order for you to remove staples or sutures, document:

- date and time the sutures were removed
- appearance of the suture line
- appearance of the wound site, including the presence of purulent drainage
- whether you notified the physician and when
- whether you collected a specimen and sent it to the laboratory for analysis and when.

TUBE FEEDINGS

When documenting your care of a patient receiving tube feedings, record:

- patient's tolerance of the procedure and the feeding formula
- type of tube feeding the patient is receiving (such as duodenal or jejunal feedings or a continuous drip or bolus)
- amount, rate, route, and method of feeding (with continuous feedings, document the rate hourly)
- dilution strength if you need to dilute the formula (for example, half-strength or three-quarter strength)
- time you flushed the tube and the type and amount of solution used, if applicable
- time you replaced the tube and how the patient tolerated the procedure, if applicable
- amount of gastric residual, if any
- description of the patient's gastric function, including prescribed medications or treatments to relieve constipation or diarrhea
- urine and serum glucose, serum electrolyte, and blood urea nitrogen levels as well as serum osmolality values
- feeding complications, such as hyperglycemia, glycosuria, and diarrhea
- patient and family teaching if the patient will continue receiving tube feedings after discharge
- referrals to suppliers or support agencies.

OBTAINING AN ARTERIAL BLOOD SAMPLE

When you obtain blood for ABG analysis, record:

- patient's vital signs and temperature
- arterial puncture site
- results of Allen's test
- indications of circulatory impairment, such as swelling, discoloration, pain, numbness, or tingling in the bandaged arm or leg, and bleeding at the puncture site
- time you drew the blood sample
- how long you applied pressure to the site to control bleeding
- type and amount of oxygen therapy the patient was receiving, if applicable.

When filling out a laboratory request form for ABG analysis, include:

- patient's current temperature and respiratory rate
- his most recent hemoglobin level
- fraction of inspired oxygen and tidal volume if he's receiving mechanical ventilation.

Assisted procedures

When you assist a physician during a procedure, you have the added responsibilities of providing patient support and teaching, evaluating the patient's response, and carefully documenting the procedure. Regardless of the procedure, you must always document:

- date, time, and name of the procedure
- physician who performed it
- how it was performed
- how the patient tolerated it
- adverse reactions to the procedure, if any
- any teaching provided to the patient.

The following section describes documentation for several procedures during which you may assist the physician.

BONE MARROW ASPIRATION

After assisting the physician with bone marrow aspiration, document:

- date and time of the procedure
- name of the physician performing the procedure
- appearance of the specimen aspirated
- how the patient responded to the procedure
- location and appearance of the aspiration site, including bleeding and drainage
- patient's vital signs after the procedure
- teaching provided to the patient.

ESOPHAGEAL TUBE INSERTION AND REMOVAL

After assisting with esophageal tube insertion or removal, document:

- date and time you assisted in the insertion or removal
- name of the physician who performed the procedure
- intragastric balloon pressure, the amount of air injected into the gastric balloon port, the amount of fluid used for gastric irrigation, and the color, consistency, and amount of gastric return before and after lavage, if applicable
- baseline intraesophageal balloon pressure, which varies with respirations and esophageal contractions
- patient's tolerance of the insertion and removal procedures
- vital signs before, during, and after the procedure.

ARTERIAL LINE INSERTION AND REMOVAL

When assisting the physician who is inserting an arterial line, record:

- date and time
- physician's name
- insertion site
- type, gauge, and length of the catheter
- patient's response to the procedure, including circulation to the involved extremity.

After removing the arterial line, record:

- date and time
- physician's name
- length of the catheter
- condition of the insertion site
- specimens that were obtained from the catheter for culture
- patient's response to the procedure
- amount of time pressure was applied at the site.

CHART QUICK

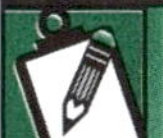

Documenting assistance during CV line insertion

The sample progress note shown below is an example of how to document when you assist in the procedure of a central venous (CV) line insertion.

Date	Time	Sign entries
6/6/02	1030	Procedure explained to pt and consent obtained by Dr. Rafferty. Triple-
		lumen catheter placed by Dr. Rafferty on 2nd attempt in Ⓛ subclavian.
		Catheter sutured in place and dressing applied as per protocol. All lines
		flushed with 5 ml NSS. Portable chest X-ray obtained to confirm place-
		ment. Pt tolerated procedure well. Vital signs stable. —— Eva Ryan, RN

CENTRAL VENOUS LINE INSERTION AND REMOVAL

When you help the physician insert a central venous (CV) line, you need to document:

- date and time of insertion
- physician's name
- length and location of the catheter
- solution infused
- patient's response to the procedure
- time that X-rays were done to confirm correct placement, the results, and when you notified the physician of them. Also document if more than one attempt was made to insert the catheter. (See *Documenting assistance during CV line insertion*.)

After assisting with removal of a CV line, record:

- date and time of removal
- type of dressing applied
- condition of the insertion site
- catheter specimens you collected for culture or other analysis.

LUMBAR PUNCTURE

During a lumbar puncture, observe the patient closely for signs of complications, such as a change in LOC, dizziness, or changes in vital signs. Report these to the physician immediately and document them carefully.

Also document:

- color and clarity of the fluid obtained
- number of test tubes sent to the laboratory for analysis
- how the patient tolerated the procedure
- observations about the patient's condition and your interventions, including keeping him in a supine position for 6 to 12 hours, encouraging fluid intake, and assessing for headache and leaking cerebrospinal fluid around the puncture site.

PARACENTESIS

When caring for a patient during and after paracentesis, document:

- date and time of the procedure
- puncture site
- whether the site was sutured
- amount, color, viscosity, and odor of the initially aspirated fluid (also, record this in the intake and output record).

If you're responsible for ongoing patient care, document:

- running record of the patient's vital signs
- frequency of drainage checks per facility protocol
- patient's response to the paracentesis
- characteristics of the drainage, including color, amount, odor, and viscosity
- patient's daily weight and abdominal girth measurements (taken at about the same time every day)
- what fluid specimens were sent to the laboratory for analysis
- peritoneal fluid leakage, if any. (Be sure to notify the physician and document the time and date.)

THORACENTESIS

When assisting with thoracentesis, you need to document:

- date and time of the procedure
- physician's name
- amount and characteristics of fluid aspirated
- patient's response to the procedure
- whether the patient had sudden or unusual pain, faintness, dizziness, or changes in vital signs and when you reported these problems to the physician
- symptoms of pneumothorax, hemothorax, subcutaneous emphysema, or infection as well as when you reported them to the physician along with your interventions
- when you sent a fluid specimen to the laboratory for analysis.

Miscellaneous procedures

Documentation isn't limited to procedures you perform or help the physician perform. You'll also document in other situations, including the ones described here.

DIAGNOSTIC TESTS

Before receiving a diagnosis, most patients undergo testing, which can be as simple as a blood test or as complicated as magnetic resonance imaging. Record in the medical record all tests and how the patient tolerated them.

Start your documentation by recording preliminary assessments you made of the patient's condition. For example, document whether she's pregnant or has allergies because these conditions might affect the way a test is performed or the test's result. If the patient's age, illness, or disability requires special preparation for a test, record this information as well.

Also document what you taught the patient about the test and follow-up care, the administration or withholding of drugs and preparations, special diets, food or fluid restrictions, enemas, and specimen collection.

PAIN CONTROL

In your quest to eliminate or minimize your patient's pain, you may use a number of assessment tools to determine the degree of pain. When you use these tools, always document the results. (See *Assessing and documenting pain.*)

When documenting pain levels and characteristics, determine whether the

CHART QUICK

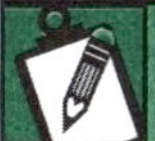

Assessing and documenting pain

Some facilities use standardized questionnaires, such as the McGill-Melzack Pain Questionnaire or the Initial Pain Assessment Tool. Alternatively, your institution may develop its own pain assessment tool, such as the flow sheet and rating scales shown below. Whichever pain assessment tool you choose, remember to document its use and put the graphic form in your patient's chart.

PAIN FLOW SHEET

Date and time	Pain rating (0 to 10)	Patient behaviors	Vital signs	Pain rating after intervention	Interventions
6/10/02 0800	7	Wincing, holding head	BP 186/88 HR 98 – RR 22	5	Dilaudid 2 mg I.M. given
6/10/02 1200	3	Relaxing, reading	BP 160/80 HR 84 – RR 18	2	

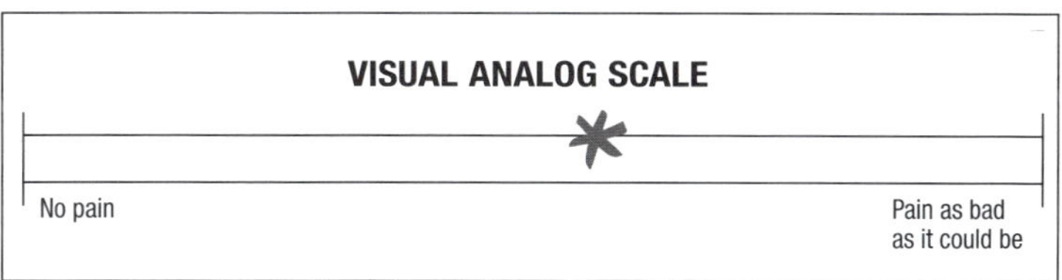

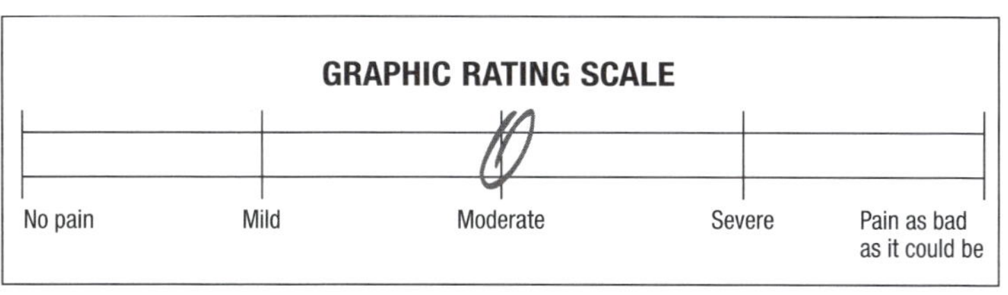

pain is internal, external, localized, or diffuse, and whether it interferes with the patient's sleep or other activities of daily living. Describe the pain in the patient's own words and enter them in the chart.

Be aware of the patient's body language and behaviors associated with pain. Does he wince or grimace? Does he move or squirm in bed? What positions seem to relieve or worsen the pain? What other measures — such as heat, cold, massage, or drugs—relieve or heighten the pain? Also, note if the pain appears to worsen or improve when visitors are present. Document all of this information as well as your interventions and how the patient responded.

INTAKE AND OUTPUT

Many patients, including surgical and burn patients, those receiving I.V. therapy, and those with fluid and electrolyte imbalances, hemorrhage, or edema need 24-hour intake and output monitoring. To expedite documentation, you'll probably keep intake and output sheets at the bedside or by the bathroom door. If the patient is incontinent, document this as well as tube drainage and irrigation volumes.

Keeping track of foods and fluids that are premeasured is easy. You can list the volumes of specific containers for quick reference and use infusion devices to more accurately record enteral and I.V. intake.

Keeping track of intake that isn't premeasured is more difficult. For example, measuring and recording a food like gelatin that's fluid at room temperature requires the cooperation of the patient and other caregivers. You'll also need to teach family members and friends to record or report to you all snacks and soft drinks they bring the patient and all meals they help him eat.

Don't forget to document as intake I.V. piggyback infusions, drugs given by I.V. push, patient-controlled analgesics, and irrigation solutions that aren't withdrawn. Also document oral or I.V. fluids that the patient receives when he isn't on your unit. This requires the cooperation of the patient and staff members in other departments. In addition, remind ambulatory patients to use a urinal or a commode.

Fluid loss through the GI tract is normally 100 ml or less daily. However, if the patient's stools become excessive or watery, you must document them as output. Vomiting, drainage from suction devices and wound drains, and bleeding are other measurable sources of fluid loss that require documentation.

TRANSFERRING A PATIENT TO A SPECIALTY UNIT

If your patient's condition deteriorates and he requires transfer to a specialty unit, make sure you record:

- date and time of the transfer as well as the name of the unit receiving the patient
- that you received transfer orders
- patient's condition at the time of transfer, including vital signs, descriptions of incisions and wounds, and locations of any tubes or medical devices still in place as well as any significant events during the hospital stay, noting whether the patient has an advance directive and other special factors, such as allergies, special diet, sensory deficits, and language or cultural issues
- medications, treatments, and teaching needs, noting which goals were and weren't met
- time that you gave a report to the receiving unit, and include the name of the nurse who received the report
- how the patient was transported to the specialty unit along with who accompanied him
- any patient teaching related to the transfer such as the reason for transfer. (Some facilities may use a transfer form to record this information.)

TERMINATING LIFE SUPPORT

According to the right-to-die laws of most states, a patient has the right to refuse extraordinary life-supporting measures if he has no hope of recovery. If the patient can't make the decision, the patient's next of kin is usually permitted to decide if life support should continue. A written statement of the patient's wishes is always preferable.

Because of the Patient Self-Determination Act, each health care facility is required to ask the patient upon admission if he has an advance directive. An advance directive is a statement of the patient's wishes if he can't make decisions for himself. An advance directive may include a living will, which goes into effect when the patient can't make decisions for himself, as well as a durable power of attorney, which names a designated person to make these decisions when the patient can't. The Act also states that the patient must receive written information concerning his right to make decisions about his medical care.

If life support is to be terminated, read the patient's advance directive to ensure that the present situation matches the patient's wishes and verify that the risk manager has reviewed the document. Check that the appropriate consent forms have been signed. Ask the family whether they would like to see the chaplain and if they would like to be with the patient before, during, and after life-support termination.

If your patient has an advance directive, you need to record:

- whether the patient's advance directive matches his present situation and life-support wishes
- that your facility's risk manager has reviewed the advance directive
- that a consent form has been signed to terminate life support, according to facility policy
- names of persons who were notified of the decision to terminate life support and their responses
- types of physical care for the patient before and after life-support termination
- whether the family was with the patient prior to, during, and after termination of life support as well as whether a chaplain was present
- time of termination, name of the physician who turned off equipment, and names of people present
- vital signs after extubation, the time the patient stopped breathing, the time he was pronounced dead, and who made the pronouncement
- family's response, your interventions for them, and after-care for the patient.

CODES

Guidelines established by the American Heart Association direct you to keep a written, chronological account of a patient's condition throughout CPR. If you're the designated recorder, document therapeutic interventions and the patient's responses as they occur. Don't rely on your memory later.

The form used to document a code is the code record. It incorporates detailed information about your observations and interventions as well as drugs given to the patient. (See *Documenting cardiopulmonary resuscitation,* pages 184 and 185.)

Some facilities use a resuscitation critique form to identify actual or potential problems with the resuscitation process. This form tracks personnel responses and response times as well as the availability of appropriate drugs

CHART QUICK

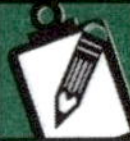

Documenting cardiopulmonary resuscitation

A completed code record like the one shown below should be included in your patient's chart.

CODE RECORD

Arrest Date: *6/21/02*
Arrest Time: *0620*
Rm/Location: *431-2*
Discovered by: *C. Brown*
☑ RN ☐ MD ☐ Other

Methods of alert:
☑ Witnessed, monitored: rhythm *V fib*
☐ Witnessed, unmonitored
☐ Unwitnessed, unmonitored
☐ Unwitnessed, monitored; rhythm

Diagnosis: *Post ant. wall MI*

Condition when needed:
☑ Unresponsive
☐ Apneic
☐ Pulseless
☐ Hemorrhage
☐ Seizure

CPR PROGRESS NOTES

Vital signs						I.V. push					Infusions			
Time	Pulse CPR	Resp. rate Spont; bag	Blood pressure	Rhythm	Defib (joules)	Atropine	Epinephrine	Lidocaine	NA bicarb	Vasopressin	Lidocaine	Procain.	Isuprel	Dopamine
0631	CPR	Bag	0	V fib			1 mg							
0632		Bag	0	V fib	200									
0633	CPR	Bag	0	A systole	300		1 mg							
0639	40	Bag	60 palp	SB PVCs				75			√			
0645	60	Bag	80/40	SB PVCs							√			

and functioning equipment. Make sure a copy of the completed critique form is submitted to the quality assurance department for analysis.

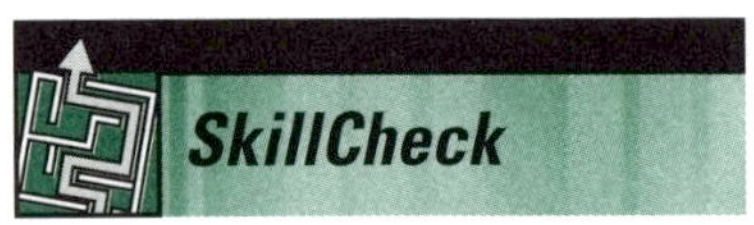

SkillCheck

1. What's one of the main purposes of an incident report?

a. To inform administrators that an

Ventilation management:
Time: 0635
Method: oral ET tube
Precordial thump: 0631
CPR initiated at: 0631

Previous airway:
☐ ET tube
☐ Trach
☑ Natural

Page. 1 of 1

Addressograph

Actions/patient response
Responses to therapy, procedures, labs drawn/results
No change
ABGs drawn Ⓡ fem pressure applied
No change
Oral intubation by Dr. Hart
CCU ready for patient

Time Spec Sent	ABGs & Lab Data						
	pH	PCO	Po_2	HCO_3	Sat%	FIO_2	Other
0633	7.1	76	43	14	80%		

RESUSCITATION OUTCOME

☑ Successful ☑ Transferred to CCU at 0648
☐ Unsuccessful – Expired at
Pronounced by: ______ MD
Family notified by: S. Quinn, RN
Time: 0645

Attending notified by:
S. Quinn, RN Time 0645
Code Recorder B. Mullen, RN
Code Team Nurse J. Hanna, RN
Anesthesia Rep. Dr. Hart
Other Personnel B. Russo, RT

incident occurred so they can take steps to prevent a recurrence.

b. To serve as proof that the incident took place.
c. To name those responsible for the incident.
d. To prevent a liability claim.

Answer: a. In addition to informing administrators of the incident, it alerts them and the facility's insurance company to a potential claim and the need for further investigation.

2. When you complete an incident report, make sure you:

a. file it in the patient's medical record.
b. note in the medical record that you filed an incident report.
c. consult a lawyer.
d. include details about the incident in your progress note.

Answer: d. There should be no mention of the incident report in the patient's medical record. However, all the details of the incident should be in your progress note.

3. Informed consent requires all of the following except:

a. description of the risks the treatment poses.
b. explanation of the consequences of refusing treatment.
c. confirmation that the patient is legally competent to give informed consent.
d. explanation that consent can't be withdrawn after it has been given.

Answer: d. The patient can always withdraw his consent after giving it.

4. If the patient develops a blood transfusion reaction, what should be your first step?

a. Notify the physician.
b. Stop the transfusion immediately.
c. Obtain blood samples as ordered by the physician.
d. Document the patient's adverse reactions.

Answer: b. You should do all of the above in the event a patient has a blood transfusion reaction; however, your first step should be to stop the transfusion as soon as possible.

5. When documenting a procedure you assisted the physician in performing, it's important to document:

a. only what you did during the procedure.
b. what you think the physician did during the procedure.
c. name of the physician who performed the procedure.
d. how you would do the procedure.

Answer: c. In addition, you should record how the patient tolerated the procedure, any adverse reactions to the procedure, and any teaching provided to the patient.

Appendices, selected references, and index

Appendix A: Commonly accepted abbreviations

Abbreviation	Meaning
AAA	abdominal aortic aneurysm
ABC	airway, breathing, circulation
ABG	arterial blood gas
a.c.	before meals
AC	assist control
ACE	angiotensin-converting enzyme
ACh	acetylcholine
ACLS	advanced cardiac life support
A.D.	auris dextra (right ear)
ADA	American Diabetes Association
ADH	antidiuretic hormone
ADLs	activities of daily living
AFIB	atrial fibrillation
AFL	atrial flutter
AFP	alpha-fetoprotein
A-G	albumin-globulin (ratio)
AHF	antihemophilic factor (factor VIII)
AICD	automatic implantable cardioverter-defibrillator
AIDS	acquired immunodeficiency syndrome
ALL	acute lymphocytic leukemia
ALS	amyotrophic lateral sclerosis
ALT	alanine aminotransferase
a.m.	morning
AMA	against medical advice American Medical Association
AMI	acute myocardial infarction
AML	acute myelocytic leukemia
amt.	amount
ANA	American Nurses Association antinuclear antibody
AP	apical pulse
APTT	activated partial thromboplastin time
ara-A	adenine arabinoside (vidarabine)
ara-C	cytosine arabinoside (cytarabine)
ARDS	acute respiratory distress syndrome
ARF	acute renal failure acute respiratory failure
AS	aortic stenosis
As	astigmatism
A.S.	auris sinistra (left ear)
ASA	acetylsalicylic acid (aspirin)
ASD	atrial septal defect
ASO	antistreptolysin-O
AST	aspartate aminotransferase
ATP	adenosine triphosphate
A.U.	each ear
AV	arteriovenous atrioventricular
AVM	arteriovenous malformation
BBB	bundle-branch block
B.B.B.	blood-brain barrier
BBT	basal body temperature

Abbreviation	Meaning
BCG	bacille Calmette-Guérin
BE	barium enema
b.i.d.	twice daily
BLS	basic life support
BM	bowel movement
BMR	basal metabolic rate
BP	blood pressure
BPH	benign prostatic hyperplasia (or hypertrophy)
BPM	beats per minute
BRB	bright red blood
BRP	bathroom privileges
BSA	body surface area
BUN	blood urea nitrogen
C	Celsius centigrade
CA	chronological age
CABG	coronary artery bypass grafting
CAD	coronary artery disease
cAMP	cyclic adenosine monophosphate
CAPD	continuous ambulatory peritoneal dialysis
caps	capsules
CBC	complete blood count
CBF	cerebral blood flow
cc	cubic centimeter
C.C.	chief complaint
CCNU	lomustine
CCU	cardiac care unit
CDC	Centers for Disease Control and Prevention
CEA	carcinoembryonic antigen
CF	cystic fibrosis
CFS	chronic fatigue syndrome
CGL	chronic granulocytic leukemia
CH	crown-heel
CHB	complete heart block
CHD	childhood disease congenital heart disease congenital hip disease
CK	creatine kinase
CK-BB	creatine kinase, brain
CK-MB	creatine kinase, heart
CK-MM	creatine kinase, skeletal muscle
cm	centimeter
CML	chronic myelogenous leukemia
CMV	cytomegalovirus
CNS	central nervous system
CO	cardiac output
c/o	complains of
comp	compound
COPD	chronic obstructive pulmonary disease
CP	capillary pressure cerebral palsy cor pulmonale creatine phosphate
CPK	creatine phosphokinase
CPAP	continuous positive airway pressure
cpm	counts per minute cycles per minute
CPR	cardiopulmonary resuscitation
CR	crown-rump
CRIS	controlled-release infusion system
C & S	culture and sensitivity
CSF	cerebrospinal fluid
CT	chest tube clotting time computed tomography
CV	cardiovascular central venous
CVA	cerebrovascular accident

Abbreviation	Meaning
CVP	central venous pressure
CXR	chest X-ray
d	day
/d	per day
D	dextrose
dB	decibel
D/C	discharge discontinue
D & C	dilatation and curettage
DD	differential diagnosis discharge diagnosis dry dressing
D & E	dilatation and evacuation
DES	diethylstilbestrol
D & I	dry and intact
DIC	disseminated intravascular coagulation
dil	dilute
disp	dispense
DJD	degenerative joint disease
DKA	diabetic ketoacidosis
dl	deciliter
DM	diabetes mellitus
DNA	deoxyribonucleic acid
DNR	do not resuscitate
D_5½NSS	dextrose 5% in 0.45% normal saline solution
DOA	date of admission dead on arrival
DS	double-strength
DSA	digital subtraction angiography
DSM-IV TR	*Diagnostic and Statistical Manual of Mental Disorders,* 4th ed., Text Revision
DTP	diphtheria and tetanus toxoids and pertussis vaccine
DTR	deep tendon reflexes
DVT	deep vein thrombosis
D_5W	dextrose 5% in water
EBV	Epstein-Barr virus
EC	enteric-coated
ECF	extracellular fluid
ECG	electrocardiogram
ECHO	echocardiography
ECMO	extracorporeal membrane oxygenator
ECT	electroconvulsive therapy
ED	emergency department
EDTA	ethylenediaminetetra-acetic acid
EEG	electroencephalogram
EENT	eyes, ears, nose, throat
EF	ejection fraction
ELISA	enzyme-linked immunosorbent assay
elix.	elixir
EMG	electromyography
EMIT	enzyme-multiplied immunoassay technique
ENG	electronystagmography
EOM	extraocular movement
ER	emergency room expiratory reserve
ERCP	endoscopic retrograde cholangiopancreatography
ERV	expiratory reserve volume
ESR	erythrocyte sedimentation rate
ESWL	extracorporeal shock-wave lithotripsy
et	and
ETT	endotracheal tube
ext.	extract
F	Fahrenheit

Abbreviation	Meaning
FDA	Food and Drug Administration
FEF	forced expiratory flow
FEV	forced expiratory volume
FFP	fresh frozen plasma
FHR	fetal heart rate
fl., fld.	fluid
Fr.	French
FRC	functional residual capacity
FSH	follicle-stimulating hormone
FSP	fibrinogen-split products
FT_3	free triiodothyronine
FT_4	free thyroxine
FTA	fluorescent treponemal antibody (test)
FTA-ABS	fluorescent treponemal antibody absorption (test)
FUO	fever of undetermined origin
FVC	forced vital capacity
G	gauge
g, gm, GM	gram
GFR	glomerular filtration rate
GI	gastrointestinal
G6PD	glucose-6-phosphate dehydrogenase
gr	grain (about 60 mg)
gt.	gutta (drop)
GU	genitourinary
GVHD	graft-versus-host disease
GYN	gynecologic
h., hr.	hour
H	hypodermic injection
HBD	alpha-hydroxybutyrate dehydrogenase
HBIG	hepatitis B immunoglobulin
HBsAg	hepatitis B surface antigen
hCG	human chorionic gonadotropin
Hct	hematocrit
HDL	high-density lipoprotein
HDN	hemolytic disease of the newborn
heme+	Hematest positive
heme–	Hematest negative
HF	heart failure
Hgb	hemoglobin
hGH	human growth hormone
HIV	human immunodeficiency virus
HLA	human leukocyte antigen
HMO	health maintenance organization
HNKS	hyperosmolar nonketotic syndrome
HOB	head of bed
hPL	human placental lactogen
h.s.	at bedtime
HS	half-strength hour of sleep house surgeon
HSV	herpes simplex virus
HVA	homovanillic acid
Hz	hertz
HZV	herpes zoster virus
IA	internal auditory intra-arterial intra-articular
IABP	intra-aortic balloon pump
IC	inspiratory capacity
ICF	intracellular fluid
ICHD	Inter-Society Commission for Heart Disease
ICP	intracranial pressure

Abbreviation	Meaning
ICU	intensive care unit
ID	identification initial dose
I & D	incision and drainage
IgM	immunoglobulin
IM	infectious mononucleosis
I.M.	intramuscular
IMV	intermittent mandatory ventilation
in.	inch
IND	investigational new drug
I/O	intake and output
IPPB	intermittent positive-pressure breathing
IRV	inspiratory reserve volume
IU	International Unit
IUD	intrauterine device
I.V.	intravenous
IVGTT	intravenous glucose tolerance test
IVH	intravenous hyperalimentation (now called total parenteral nutrition [TPN])
IVP	intravenous pyelography
IVPB	intravenous piggyback
J	joule
JCAHO	Joint Commission on Accreditation of Healthcare Organizations
JP	Jackson-Pratt (drain)
JVD	jugular venous distention
JVP	jugular venous pressure
kg	kilogram
17-KGS	17-ketogenic steroids
17-KS	17-ketosteroids
KUB	kidney-ureter-bladder
KVO	keep vein open
L	liter lumbar
LA	left atrium long-acting
LAP	left atrial pressure leucine aminopeptidase
lb	pound
LBBB	left bundle-branch block
LD	lactate dehydrogenase
LDL	low-density lipoprotein
LE	lupus erythematosus
LES	lower esophageal sphincter
LGL	Lown-Ganong-Levine variant syndrome
LH	luteinizing hormone
LLL	left lower leg left lower lobe
LLQ	left lower quadrant
L/min	liters per minute
LOC	level of consciousness
LR	lactated Ringer's solution
LSB	left scapular border left sternal border
LSC	left subclavian
LTC	long-term care
LUQ	left upper quadrant
LV	left ventricle
LVEDP	left ventricular end-diastolic pressure
LVET	left ventricular ejection time
LVF	left ventricular failure
m	meter
M	molar (solution)
m^2	square meter
MAO	monoamine oxidase
MAR	medication administration record

Abbreviation	Meaning
MAST	medical antishock trousers (pneumatic antishock garment)
mcg	microgram
MCH	mean corpuscular hemoglobin
MCHC	mean corpuscular hemoglobin concentration
MCV	mean corpuscular volume
MD	medical doctor muscular dystrophy
mEq	milliequivalent
mg	milligram
mgtt	microdrip or minidrop
MI	mitral insufficiency myocardial infarction
ml	milliliter
µl	microliter
MLC	mixed lymphocyte culture
mm	millimeter
mm^3	cubic millimeter
MMEF	maximal midexpiratory flow
mmol	millimole
MRI	magnetic resonance imaging
M.R. × 1	may repeat once
MS	mitral stenosis morphine sulfate multiple sclerosis
MUGA	multiple-gated acquisition (scanning)
MVI	multivitamin infusion
MVP	mitral valve prolapse
MVV	maximal voluntary ventilation
NC	nasal cannula
ng	nanogram
NG	nasogastric
NICU	neonatal intensive care unit
NKA	no known allergies
NMR	nuclear magnetic resonance
Noct.	night
NPN	nonprotein nitrogen
NPO	nothing by mouth
NR	nonreactive
N/R	not remarkable
NS, NSS	normal saline solution (0.9% sodium chloride solution)
¼ NS	¼ normal saline solution (0.225% sodium chloride solution)
½ NS	½ normal saline solution (0.45% sodium chloride solution)
NSAID	nonsteroidal anti-inflammatory drug
NSR	normal sinus rhythm
N/V	nausea and vomiting
OB	obstetric
OD	oculus dexter (right eye) overdose
OGTT	oral glucose tolerance test
OOB	out of bed
OR	operating room
OS	oculus sinister (left eye)
OTC	over-the-counter
OU	oculus uterque (each eye)
oz	ounce
P	pulse
PA	posteroanterior pulmonary artery
PABA	para-aminobenzoic acid
PAC	premature atrial contraction
$Paco_2$	partial pressure of arterial carbon dioxide

Abbreviation	Meaning
PACU	postanesthesia care unit
Pao_2	partial pressure of arterial oxygen
Pap	Papanicolaou smear
PAP	pulmonary artery pressure
PAT	paroxysmal atrial tachycardia
PAWP	pulmonary artery wedge pressure
p.c.	after meals
PCA	patient-controlled analgesia
PC X-ray	portable chest X-ray
PDA	patent ductus arteriosus
PE	physical examination pulmonary embolism
PEARL	pupils equal and reactive to light
PEEP	positive end-expiratory pressure
PEFR	peak expiratory flow rate
PEP	preejection period
per	by or through
PET	positron emission tomography
pg	picogram
PICC	peripherally inserted central catheter
PID	pelvic inflammatory disease
PKU	phenylketonuria
p.m.	afternoon
PMI	point of maximum impulse
PML	progressive multifocal leukoencephalopathy
PMS	premenstrual syndrome
PND	paroxysmal nocturnal dyspnea postnasal drip
P.O.	by mouth
PP	partial pressure peripheral pulses
PR	by rectum
PRBC	packed red blood cells
p.r.n.	as needed
PROM	passive range of motion premature rupture of the membranes
pt., Pt.	patient
PT	pint prothrombin time
PTCA	percutaneous transluminal coronary angioplasty
PTH	parathyroid hormone
PTT	partial thromboplastin time
PUD	peptic ulcer disease
PVC	polyvinyl chloride premature ventricular contraction
q	every
q a.m.	every morning
q.d.	every day
q.h.	every hour
q.i.d.	four times daily
q.n.	every night
q.o.d.	every other day
QS	quantity sufficient
qt.	quart
R	by rectum respiration
RA	rheumatoid arthritis right atrium
RAF	rheumatoid arthritis factor
RAP	right atrial pressure
RAST	radioallergosorbent test
RBBB	right bundle-branch block
RBC	red blood cell

Abbreviation	Meaning
RDA	recommended daily allowance
RE	rectal examination
REM	rapid eye movement
RES	reticuloendothelial system
Rh	rhesus blood factor
RHD	rheumatic heart disease
RIA	radioimmunoassay
RL	right lateral
RLQ	Ringer's lactate (lactated Ringer's solution) right lower quadrant
RNA	ribonucleic acid
R/O	rule out
ROM	range of motion rupture of membranes
RR	respiratory rate
RRR	regular rate and rhythm
RSC	right subclavian
RSV	respiratory syncytial virus right subclavian vein Rous sarcoma virus
R/T	related to
RUQ	right upper quadrant
RV	residual volume right ventricle
RVEDP	right ventricular end-diastolic pressure
RVEDV	right ventricular end-diastolic volume
RVP	right ventricular pressure
Rx	prescription
SA	sinoatrial
Sao_2	arterial oxygen saturation
sat.	saturated
SC	subclavian
S.C., SQ	subcutaneous
SCID	severe combined immunodeficiency syndrome
sec	second
SGOT	serum glutamic-oxaloacetic transaminase (now called aspartate aminotransferase [AST])
SGPT	serum glutamic-pyruvic transaminase (now called alanineaminotransferase [ALT])
SHBG	sex hormone-binding globulin
SI	Système International d'Unités (International System of Units)
SIADH	syndrome of inappropriate antidiuretic hormone
SIDS	sudden infant death syndrome
Sig	write on label
SIMV	synchronized intermittent mandatory ventilation
SLE	systemic lupus erythematosus
SOB	shortness of breath
sol., soln.	solution
SR	sustained release
SRS-A	slow-reacting substance of anaphylaxis
stat	immediately
STD	sexually transmitted disease
supp	suppository
susp	suspension
SV	stroke volume
$S\bar{v}o_2$	mixed venous oxygen saturation
syr.	syrup
T	temperature

Abbreviation	Meaning
T, Tbs, tbsp	tablespoon
t, tsp	teaspoon
tab	tablet
TBG	thyroxine-binding globulin
TCA	tricyclic antidepressant
TENS	transcutaneous electrical nerve stimulation
TIA	transient ischemic attack
t.i.d.	three times daily
TIL	tumor-infiltrating lymphocyte
tinct., tr.	tincture
TLC	total lung capacity triple lumen catheter
TM	temporomandibular tympanic membrane
TMJ	temporomandibular joint
TNF	tumor necrosis factor
TO	telephone order
tol.	tolerate tolerates tolerated
tPA	tissue plasminogen activator
TPN	total parenteral nutrition
TRH	thyrotropin-releasing hormone
TSH	thyroid-stimulating hormone
UA	urinalysis
UCE	urea cycle enzymopathy
USP	United States Pharmacopeia
UTI	urinary tract infection
UV	ultraviolet
V, vag.	vaginal
VAD	vascular access device ventricular assist device
VAP	vascular access port
VDRL	Venereal Disease Research Laboratory (test)
VLDL	very low density lipoprotein
VMA	vanillylmandelic acid
VO	verbal order
$\dot{V}/\dot{Q}$	ventilation-perfusion ratio
VS	vital signs
VSD	ventricular septal defect
VSS	vital signs stable
V_T, Vt	tidal volume
WBC	white blood cell
WNL	within normal limits
w/o	without
WPW	Wolff-Parkinson-White syndrome
Z/G, ZIG	zoster immune globulin

Appendix B: Commonly accepted symbols

Symbol	Meaning
Pulses	
0	absent; impalpable
+1	weak or thready; hard to feel; easily obliterated by slight finger pressure
+2	normal; easily palpable; obliterated only by strong finger pressure
+3	bounding; readily palpable; forceful; not easily obliterated
Reflexes	
+ + + +	very brisk; hyperactive
+ + +	increased, but not necessarily abnormal
+ +	average; normal
+	present, but diminished
0	absent
Heart murmurs	
1/6 or I/VI	faint; barely audible even to the trained ear; may not be heard in all positions
2/6 or II/VI	soft and low; easily audible to the trained ear
3/6 or III/VI	moderately loud; approximately equal to the intensity of normal heart sounds
4/6 or IV/VI	very loud, with a palpable thrill at the murmur site
5/6 or V/VI	very loud, with a palpable thrill; audible with stethoscope in partial contact with chest
6/6 or VI/VI	extremely loud, with a palpable thrill; audible with stethoscope over but not in contact with chest

Symbol	Meaning
Apothecary symbols	
♏	minim (about 0.06 ml)
℞	prescription
ʒ	dram
℥	ounce
Other symbols	
ā	before
āā	each
@	at
c̄	with
Ca	calcium
Cl	chloride
CO	cardiac output, carbon monoxide
CO_2	carbon dioxide
Hg	mercury
K	potassium
Ⓛ	left
(LA)	left arm
(LL)	left leg
Na	sodium
NaCl	sodium chloride
O_2	oxygen
Ⓡ	right
(RA)	right arm
(RL)	right leg
♀	female
♂	male
′	foot, feet
″	inch, inches
#	number, pound

Symbol	Meaning	Symbol	Meaning
Other symbols (continued)		**Other symbols** (continued)	
+	excess, plus, positive	↓	decrease
–	deficiency, minus, negative	?	questionable
>	greater than	ø, ȱ	none, no
≥	greater than or equal to	1°	primary, first degree
<	less than	2°	secondary, second degree
≤	less than or equal to	3°	tertiary, third degree
Λ	diastolic blood pressure (commonly used on graphic forms)	1:1	one-to-one
V	systolic blood pressure	p̄	after
≅	approximately equal to	s̄	without
≈	approximately	ss, s̄s̄, ṡṡ	one-half
↑	increase	×	times
		i̇̄	one
		ï̄	two

Appendix C: NANDA Taxonomy II codes

The North American Nursing Diagnosis Association (NANDA) endorsed its first nursing diagnosis taxonomic structure, NANDA Taxonomy I, in 1986. This taxonomy has been revised several times, most recently in 2000. The new Taxonomy II has a code structure that's compliant with the recommendations of the National Library of Medicine concerning health care terminology codes. The taxonomy that appears here represents the accepted classification system for nursing diagnosis.

Taxonomy II codes	Nursing diagnosis
00001	Imbalanced nutrition: More than body requirements
00002	Imbalanced nutrition: Less than body requirements
00003	Risk for imbalanced nutrition: More than body requirements
00004	Risk for infection
00005	Risk for imbalanced body temperature
00006	Hypothermia
00007	Hyperthermia
00008	Ineffective thermoregulation
00009	Autonomic dysreflexia
00010	Risk for autonomic dysreflexia
00011	Constipation
00012	Perceived constipation
00013	Diarrhea
00014	Bowel incontinence
00015	Risk for constipation
00016	Impaired urinary elimination
00017	Stress urinary incontinence
00018	Reflex urinary incontinence
00019	Urge urinary incontinence
00020	Functional urinary incontinence
00021	Total urinary incontinence
00022	Risk for urge urinary incontinence
00023	Urinary retention
00024	Ineffective tissue perfusion (specify type: renal, cerebral, cardiopulmonary, gastrointestinal, peripheral)
00025	Risk for imbalanced fluid volume
00026	Excess fluid volume
00027	Deficient fluid volume
00028	Risk for deficient fluid volume
00029	Decreased cardiac output
00030	Impaired gas exchange
00031	Ineffective airway clearance
00032	Ineffective breathing pattern
00033	Impaired spontaneous ventilation
00034	Dysfunctional ventilatory weaning response
00035	Risk for injury
00036	Risk for suffocation
00037	Risk for poisoning
00038	Risk for trauma
00039	Risk for aspiration
00040	Risk for disuse syndrome
00041	Latex allergy response

Taxonomy II codes	Nursing diagnosis	Taxonomy II codes	Nursing diagnosis
00042	Risk for latex allergy response	00073	Disabled family coping
00043	Ineffective protection	00074	Compromised family coping
00044	Impaired tissue integrity	00075	Readiness for enhanced family coping
00045	Impaired oral mucous membrane	00076	Readiness for enhanced community coping
00046	Impaired skin integrity	00077	Ineffective community coping
00047	Risk for impaired skin integrity	00078	Ineffective therapeutic regimen management
00048	Impaired dentition	00079	Noncompliance (specify)
00049	Decreased intracranial adaptive capacity	00080	Ineffective family therapeutic regimen management
00050	Disturbed energy field	00081	Ineffective community therapeutic regimen management
00051	Impaired verbal communication	00082	Effective therapeutic regimen management
00052	Impaired social interaction	00083	Decisional conflict (specify)
00053	Social isolation	00084	Health-seeking behaviors (specify)
00054	Risk for loneliness	00085	Impaired physical mobility
00055	Ineffective role performance	00086	Risk for peripheral neurovascular dysfunction
00056	Impaired parenting	00087	Risk for perioperative-positioning injury
00057	Risk for impaired parenting	00088	Impaired walking
00058	Risk for impaired parent/infant/child attachment	00089	Impaired wheelchair mobility
00059	Sexual dysfunction	00090	Impaired transfer ability
00060	Interrupted family processes	00091	Impaired bed mobility
00061	Caregiver role strain	00092	Activity intolerance
00062	Risk for caregiver role strain	00093	Fatigue
00063	Dysfunctional family processes: Alcoholism	00094	Risk for activity intolerance
00064	Parental role conflict	00095	Disturbed sleep pattern
00065	Ineffective sexuality patterns	00096	Sleep deprivation
00066	Spiritual distress	00097	Deficient diversional activity
00067	Risk of spiritual distress	00098	Impaired home maintenance
00068	Readiness for enhanced spiritual well-being	00099	Ineffective health maintenance
00069	Ineffective coping	00100	Delayed surgical recovery
00070	Impaired adjustment	00101	Adult failure to thrive
00071	Defensive coping	00102	Feeding self-care deficit
00072	Ineffective denial		

Taxonomy II codes	Nursing diagnosis
00103	Impaired swallowing
00104	Ineffective breast-feeding
00105	Interrupted breast-feeding
00106	Effective breast-feeding
00107	Ineffective infant feeding pattern
00108	Bathing or hygiene self-care deficit
00109	Dressing or grooming self-care deficit
00110	Toileting self-care deficit
00111	Delayed growth and development
00112	Risk for delayed development
00113	Risk for disproportionate growth
00114	Relocation stress syndrome
00115	Risk for disorganized infant behavior
00116	Disorganized infant behavior
00117	Readiness for enhanced organized infant behavior
00118	Disturbed body image
00119	Chronic low self-esteem
00120	Situational low self-esteem
00121	Disturbed personal identity
00122	Disturbed sensory perception (specify: visual, auditory, kinesthetic, gustatory, tactile, olfactory)
00123	Unilateral neglect
00124	Hopelessness
00125	Powerlessness
00126	Deficient knowledge (specify)
00127	Impaired environmental interpretation syndrome
00128	Acute confusion
00129	Chronic confusion
00130	Disturbed thought processes
00131	Impaired memory
00132	Acute pain
00133	Chronic pain
00134	Nausea
00135	Dysfunctional grieving
00136	Anticipatory grieving
00137	Chronic sorrow
00138	Risk for other-directed violence
00139	Risk for self-mutilation
00140	Risk for self-directed violence
00141	Posttrauma syndrome
00142	Rape-trauma syndrome
00143	Rape-trauma syndrome: Compound reaction
00144	Rape-trauma syndrome: Silent reaction
00145	Risk for posttrauma syndrome
00146	Anxiety
00147	Death anxiety
00148	Fear

New nursing diagnoses: Effective April 2000

Taxonomy II codes	Nursing diagnosis
00149	Risk for relocation stress syndrome
00150	Risk for suicide
00151	Self-mutilation
00152	Risk for powerlessness
00153	Risk for situational low self-esteem
00154	Wandering
00155	Risk for falls

Selected references

ChartSmart: The A-to-Z Guide to Better Nursing Documentation. Springhouse, Pa.: Springhouse Corp., 2002.

Coty, E.L., Davis, J., and Angell, L. *Documentation: The Language of Nursing.* Upper Saddle River, N.J.: Prentice Hall, 2000.

Iyer, P.W., and Camp, N.H. *Nursing Documentation: A Nursing Process Approach,* 3rd ed. St. Louis: Mosby–Year Book, Inc., 1999.

Joint Commission on Accreditation of Healthcare Organizations (JCAHO). *Comprehensive Accreditation Manual for Hospitals: The Official Handbook.* Oakbrook Terrace, Ill.: JCAHO, 2002.

Marrelli, T.M. *Handbook of Home Health Standards and Documentation Guidelines for Reimbursement,* 4th ed. St. Louis: Mosby–Year Book, Inc., 2001.

Marrelli, T.M., and Harper, D.S. *Nursing Documentation Handbook,* 3rd ed. St. Louis: Mosby–Year Book, Inc., 2000.

Meiner, S.E. *Nursing Documentation: Legal Focus Across Practice Settings.* Thousand Oaks, Calif.: Sage Publications, 1999.

Nurse's Legal Handbook, 4th ed. Springhouse, Pa.: Springhouse Corp., 2000.

Sparks, S., and Taylor, C. *Nursing Diagnosis Reference Manual,* 5th ed., Springhouse, Pa.: Springhouse Corp., 2001.

Surefire Documentation: How, What, and When Nurses Need to Document. St. Louis: Mosby–Year Book, Inc., 1999.

Index

A

Abbreviations
- common, 188-196
- inappropriate, 41, 42-43i

Abuse, drug, 169
Accountability, 5
Accreditation, 3, 4
Action plan, 29
Activities of daily living
- assessment of, 13
  - Barthel index for, 132-133i
  - Katz index for, 129-130i
  - Lawton scale for, 131i
- in long-term care, 124

Acute care documentation, 93-115
- admission database form in, 94-97, 95-96i, 114
- care plans in, 97, 98
- critical pathways in, 97, 98
- discharge summaries in, 112-114, 113i, 114i, 115
- flow sheets in, 109, 110-111i, 114
- graphic form in, 103-107, 106i
- patient care Kardex in, 99-103, 100-101i, 102i, 104-105i, 115
- progress notes in, 107, 108i, 115

Admission assessment, 94
Admission database form, 94, 95-96i
- problems of, 97

Admissions, in home care, evaluation of, 140, 141
Advance directives, 159
- checklist for, 162, 163i
- termination of life support and, 183
- tips for dealing with, 161

Adverse events, prevention of, 59
Against-medical-advice form, 167
AIR documentation, 66
Allergic reaction, in I.V. therapy, 170
American Nurses Association, credentialing requirement of, 51
Anticipated recovery plan, 29
Arterial blood gas analysis, 177
Arterial line, insertion and removal of, 178
Aspiration, bone marrow, 178
Assessment
- in charting by exception, 77
- in FACT documentation system, 83, 84i
- health history and , 9
- in home care, 141, 145, 146-147i
- Joint Commission on Accreditation of Healthcare Organizations standards for, 12
- nursing process and, 8
- physical examination and, 11, 12
- priorities for, 15

Automated documentation. *See* Computerized documentation.

B

Balanced Budget Act, 138
Barthel index, 130, 132-133i
Bias, in documentation, 54

i refers to an illustration; t refers to a table.

Blood sample, arterial, 177
Blood transfusion reaction, 171i, 186
Blood transfusions, 170, 171i
Bone marrow aspiration, 178

C

Cardiac monitoring, 174
Cardiopulmonary resuscitation, 183, 184-185i
Cardiovascular system, assessment of, 12
Care map, 29
Care plans, 18, 22-29
  in acute care documentation, 97, 98
  aspects of, 22
  in Core documentation system, 86
  in charting by exception, 76
  creating, 19
  in home care, 145, 148i, 152i
  Joint Commission on Accreditation of Healthcare Organizations requirements for, 23
  in long-term care, 130
  revision to, 22
  standardized, 23, 24i
  traditional, 23, 24i
  types of, 23
  writing, 18, 19, 22
Care track, 98
Centers for Medicare and Medicaid Service, 117
Central venous line, insertion and removal of, 179, 179i
Chart check, 45
Charting. *See* Documentation.
Charting by exception, 64-65t, 75-83, 92
  advantages of, 79
  disadvantages of, 82
Charting by exception *(continued)*
  flow sheets in, 76, 77i, 78, 79-82i
  format and components of, 76
  don’ts of, 54, 56-57
Charts, patient requests for, 166
Chest physiotherapy, 175
Chronological documentation, 39, 41i
Clinical pathways, 29
  in acute care, 97, 98
  advantages and disadvantages of, 37
  goals of, 29
  model of, 32-37t
  prioritization in, 38
  structure of, 36
Clinical records. *See* Medical records.
Code record, 183, 184-185i
Codes, 183
Colon resection, clinical pathway for, 32-37t
Communication, documentation as, 2
Community Health Accreditation Program, 140, 145
Computerized documentation, 7, 66-67t, 87-90
  advantages and disadvantages of, 90
  confidentiality in, 153, 154, 155
  drug administration and, 168
  electronic signature in, 45
  in home care, 151
  physicians’ orders and, 45
  successful, 8
  timeliness in, 39
Computers, laptop, 151, 154
Computer systems, 87
  nursing information, 88
  voice-activated, 90
Confidentiality, 40
  in computerized documentation, 153, 154, 155

i refers to an illustration; t refers to a table.

Consent form, 158
and termination of life support, 183
witnessing, 159
Core documentation system, 86-87
Countersigning, 45, 47, 48
Critical pathways. *See* Clinical pathways.

D

Dermal drugs, 168
Dermal patches, 169
Diabetes mellitus, patient-teaching record for, 30-31i
Diagnosis-related groups, 4
Diagnostic tests, 180
Dialysis, peritoneal, 173
Discharge forms, in long-term care, 134
Discharge instructions, documentation of, 55
Discharge planning, 50
in charting by exception, 78
Discharge planning needs, as factor in assessment, 13, 14i
Discharge summary
in acute care, 112-114, 113i
in Core documentation system, 86
in home care, 150
in problem-oriented medical record, 69
Documentation
chronological, 39, 41i
computerized. *See* Computerized documentation.
confidentiality in, 39, 40
content for, 54, 55i, 56-57
delegation in, 57, 61
efficient, tips for, 6
enhancing, 38-45, 50
Documentation *(continued)*
fundamentals of, 1-50
guidelines for, 53-58
in acute care. *See* Acute care documentation.
in home care. *See* Home care documentation.
in long-term care. *See* Long-term care documentation.
in special situations, 156-186
legal aspects of, 51-61
legibility in, 40
objectivity in, 38
purposes of, 1-5
risk management and, 58-61
signature in, 44
timeliness of, 39, 57
Documentation systems, 62-92
charting by exception, 64-65t, 75-83, 77i, 79-82i, 92
choosing, 91-92
comparing, 64-67t
computerized, 66-67t, 87-90
Core, 66-67t, 86-87, 91
FACT, 64-65t, 83-86, 84-85i
FOCUS, 73-75, 74i
problem-intervention-evaluation, 64-65t, 71-73, 72i, 91
problem-oriented, 64-65t, 68-71, 70i, 91
traditional narrative, 62-68, 63i, 64-65t
Do-not-resuscitate orders, 162
Drainage, thoracic, 174
Drug abuse, 169
Drug administration, documentation of, 168
Drugs
as-needed, 168

i refers to an illustration; t refers to a table.

Drugs *(continued)*
refusal of, 169
Durable power of attorney, 162
tips for dealing with, 161

E

Eardrops, 168
Ears, assessment of, 12
Education, documentation and, 2
E-mail, and confidentiality, 153, 155
Environment, as factor in assessment, 13
Errors, correction of, 41, 44i, 49
Esophageal tube, insertion and removal of, 178
Evaluation, of interventions, 20, 21
Evaluation statements, 22
Expected outcomes, 21
evaluation of, 22
Extravasation, in I.V. therapy, 170
Eyedrops, 168
Eyes, assessment of, 12

F

FACT documentation system, 64-65t, 83-86, 84-85i
advantages of, 83
disadvantages of, 86
format and components of, 83
Family, as factor in assessment, 14
Flow sheets
activities of daily living, in long-term care, 124
in acute care documentation, 109, 110-111i
advantages of, 109
in charting by exception, 76, 77i, 78, 79-82i

Flow sheets *(continued)*
in Core documentation system, 86
disadvantages of, 111
in FACT documentation system, 83
how to use, 112
pain, 181, 181i
FOCUS documentation system, 73-75, 74i

G

Gastrointestinal system, assessment of, 12
Genitourinary system, assessment of, 12
Graphic form
in acute care documentation, 103-107, 106i
advantages of, 106
disadvantages of, 107
how to use, 107

H

Handwriting, 40
Health care, evaluation of, 2
Health history, 9, 11
nursing, 50
obtaining, 10, 11
History, medical versus nursing, 9
Home care agencies, legal responsibilities of, 140-143
Home care certification and care plan, 151, 152i
Home care documentation
assessment and, 145
evaluation of admissions in, 140, 141
and financial losses, 140
forms for, 143-151
future developments in, 151-154

i refers to an illustration; t refers to a table.

Home care documentation *(continued)*
legal risks and responsibilities in, 140-143
and liability, 140
Medicare forms in, 151, 152i, 153i, 154i
Outcome and Assessment Information Set requirements in, 138-140
patient assessment in, 139
and patient teaching, 143, 144i
referral form in, 141, 142i
Hospice services, 139

I

I.V. medications, 169
I.V. therapy, 169
Incident reports, 59, 156, 157
purpose of, 184
tips for, 158
Incidents, managing, 60
Incision, surgical, care of, 172
Informed consent, 158, 160, 186
Initial nursing assessment form, in long-term care, 118, 124
Intake and output, monitoring, 182
Integumentary system, assessment of, 12
Interdisciplinary action plan, 29
Interdisciplinary plan, 29
Interventions, 19
in charting by exception, 78
evaluation of, 20, 21
Interview, in health history, 11
Intramuscular medications, 169

J

Joint Commission on Accreditation of Healthcare Organizations, 3
Joint Commission on Accreditation of Healthcare Organizations *(continued)*
assessment standards of, 12
care plan requirements of, 23
long-term care standards of, 118

K

Kardex, 99-103
advantages of, 99
components of, 99, 100-101
computerized, 99, 102i
disadvantages of, 102
how to use, 103
medication, 103, 104-105i
Katz index, 128, 129-130i, 137

L

Language, in documentation, 54
Laptop computers, 151, 154
Last will and testament, tips for dealing with, 161
Lavage, peritoneal, 174
Lawsuits, 52, 61
Lawton scale, 130, 131i
Learning needs
as factor in assessment, 13
and patient-teaching plan, 26
Learning outcomes
and patient teaching plan, 26
writing, 27i
Legal competence, 161
Legal protection, documentation as, 2
Legal situations, documentation in, 156-167
Legibility, 40
Licensing, 3
Licensure, for home health agencies, 140

i refers to an illustration; t refers to a table.

Life support, termination of, 183
Living will, 162
tips for dealing with, 161
Long-term care, levels of, 116, 137
Long-term care documentation, 116-137
care plans in, 130
guidelines for, 134-136
regulation of, 116-118
standards and requirements for, 118-134
Lumbar puncture, 179

M

Malpractice litigation, 52, 61
Maslow's hierarchy of needs, 15, 16i
Mechanical ventilation, 175
Medicaid, in long-term care, 117
Medical records
components of, 4
in court, 51, 52
patient request for, 166
for home health care nurses, 7
problem-oriented, 6, 7i
source-oriented narrative, 6
types of, 5-8
uses for, 1
Medical update and patient information form, 151, 153i
Medicare
and hospice services, 139
in long-term care,117
and physician's telephone orders, 151, 154i
role of, in home care, 138
Medicare forms, in home care, 151, 152i, 153i, 154i
Medication administration record, 168
Medications
as-needed, 168
refusal of, 169
Military time, 39
Minimum Data Set form, in long-term care, 118, 119-123i
Monitoring
cardiac, 174
intake and output, 182
Mouth, assessment of, 12
Musculoskeletal system, assessment of, 12

N

Narcotics, administration of, 169
Narrative documentation. *See* Traditional narrative documentation.
Nasogastric tube, insertion and removal of, 176, 176i
National League for Nursing, 140
Negligence, 58, 61
incident report and, 158
Neurologic system, assessment of, 12
Nightingale, Florence, 1
North American Nursing Diagnosis Association, 14
taxonomy II codes of, 199-201
Nose, assessment of, 12
Nose drops, 168
Nurse practice acts, 5
and legal responsibilities, 51
Nursing diagnosis, 14, 16i
Nursing information systems, 88
Nursing interventions, 19
in charting by exception, 78
evaluation of, 20, 21
writing, 20

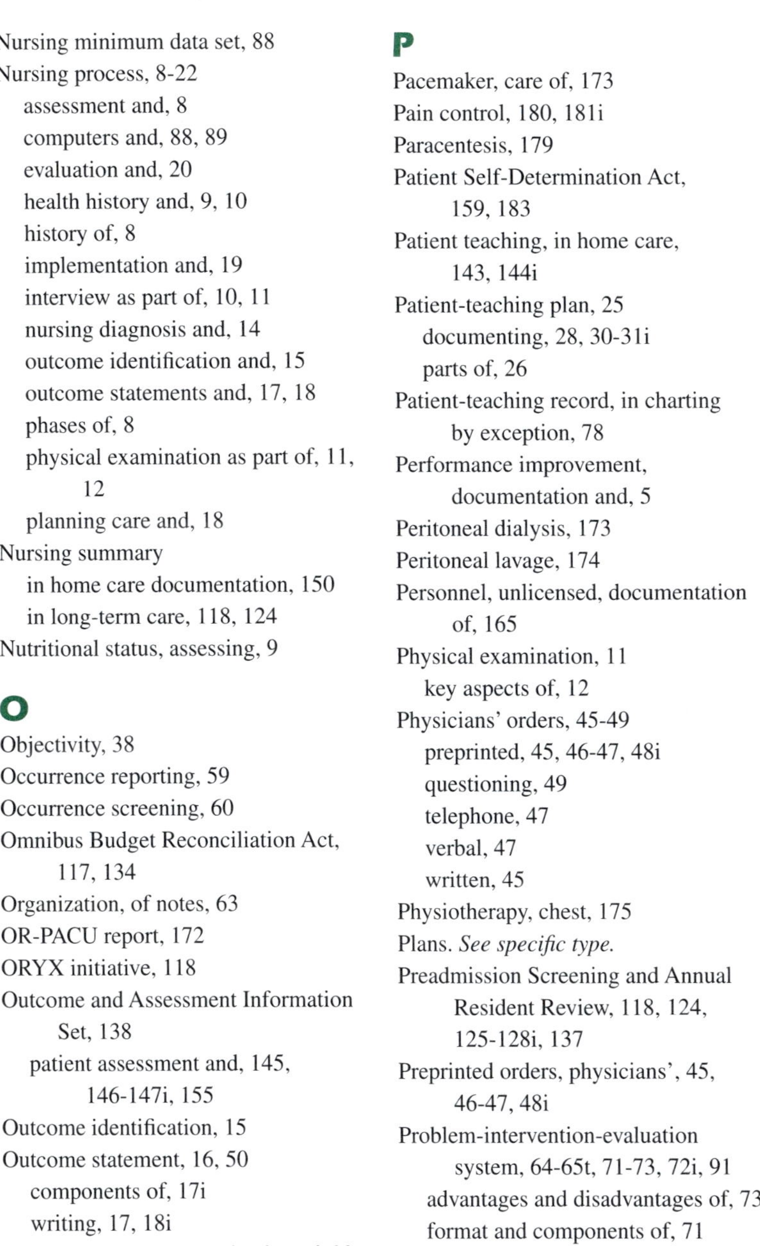

Nursing minimum data set, 88
Nursing process, 8-22
assessment and, 8
computers and, 88, 89
evaluation and, 20
health history and, 9, 10
history of, 8
implementation and, 19
interview as part of, 10, 11
nursing diagnosis and, 14
outcome identification and, 15
outcome statements and, 17, 18
phases of, 8
physical examination as part of, 11, 12
planning care and, 18
Nursing summary
in home care documentation, 150
in long-term care, 118, 124
Nutritional status, assessing, 9

O

Objectivity, 38
Occurrence reporting, 59
Occurrence screening, 60
Omnibus Budget Reconciliation Act, 117, 134
Organization, of notes, 63
OR-PACU report, 172
ORYX initiative, 118
Outcome and Assessment Information Set, 138
patient assessment and, 145, 146-147i, 155
Outcome identification, 15
Outcome statement, 16, 50
components of, 17i
writing, 17, 18i
Outcomes, expected, evaluation of, 22

P

Pacemaker, care of, 173
Pain control, 180, 181i
Paracentesis, 179
Patient Self-Determination Act, 159, 183
Patient teaching, in home care, 143, 144i
Patient-teaching plan, 25
documenting, 28, 30-31i
parts of, 26
Patient-teaching record, in charting by exception, 78
Performance improvement, documentation and, 5
Peritoneal dialysis, 173
Peritoneal lavage, 174
Personnel, unlicensed, documentation of, 165
Physical examination, 11
key aspects of, 12
Physicians' orders, 45-49
preprinted, 45, 46-47, 48i
questioning, 49
telephone, 47
verbal, 47
written, 45
Physiotherapy, chest, 175
Plans. *See specific type.*
Preadmission Screening and Annual Resident Review, 118, 124, 125-128i, 137
Preprinted orders, physicians', 45, 46-47, 48i
Problem-intervention-evaluation system, 64-65t, 71-73, 72i, 91
advantages and disadvantages of, 73
format and components of, 71

i refers to an illustration; t refers to a table.

Problem list, 7, 7i
Problem-oriented medical record, 64-65t, 68-71, 70i, 91
advantages of, 69
disadvantages of, 71
format and components of, 68
Procedures, 167-177
assisted, 178-180, 186
guidelines for, 168
Progress notes
in acute care documentation, 107, 108i
in charting by exception, 78
in Core documentation system, 86
documenting incidents in, 156
in FACT documentation system, 83
in FOCUS system, 74i, 75
in home care documentation, 149, 155
how to write, 108
in problem-oriented medical record, 69, 70i
Prospective payment system, 138, 155

Q

Quality assurance, versus risk management, 60

R

Referral form, in home care admission, 141, 142i
Refusal of treatment, 164, 164i
legal guidelines for, 165
Reimbursement, documentation and, 3
Reproductive system, assessment of, 12
Research, documentation and, 2
Resident Assessment Protocol, 118, 124, 137
Respiratory system, assessment of, 12
Restraints, use of, 166, 166i
Resuscitation critique form, 183
Right-to-die laws, 183
Risk management, 58-61
goals of, 59
managing incidents and, 60
preventing adverse events and, 59

S

Screening, in home care admission, 141
Seizures, management of, 176
Signature, 43
physician's, 47
Skin, assessment of, 12
SOAP documentation, 69, 71, 92
Specialty unit, transferring to, 182
Staples, removal of, 177
Subcutaneous medications, 169
Suppositories, 168
Surgical incision, care of, 172
Sutures, removal of, 177
Symbols, common, 197-198

T

Telephone orders, physician's, 47, 151, 154i
Thoracentesis, 180
Thoracic drainage, 174
Throat, assessment of, 12
Timeliness, 39, 57
Total parenteral nutrition, 169, 170
Traditional narrative documentation, 62-68, 63i
advantages and disadvantages of, 67
format and components of, 62
Transfer, to specialty unit, 182

i refers to an illustration; t refers to a table.

Transfer forms, in long-term care, 134, 135-136i
Transfusions, blood, 170, 171i
Treatment, refusal of, 164, 164i, 165
Tube feedings, 177
Tubes
  esophageal, insertion and removal of, 178
  nasogastric, insertion and removal of, 176, 176i

Unlicensed personnel, documentation of, 165

V

Ventilation, mechanical, 175
Verbal orders, physicians', 47
Voice-activated systems, 90

WXYZ

Wound care, postsurgical, 172
Written orders, physicians', 45

i refers to an illustration; t refers to a table.

Notes

Notes

Notes